KETO CELEBRATIONS

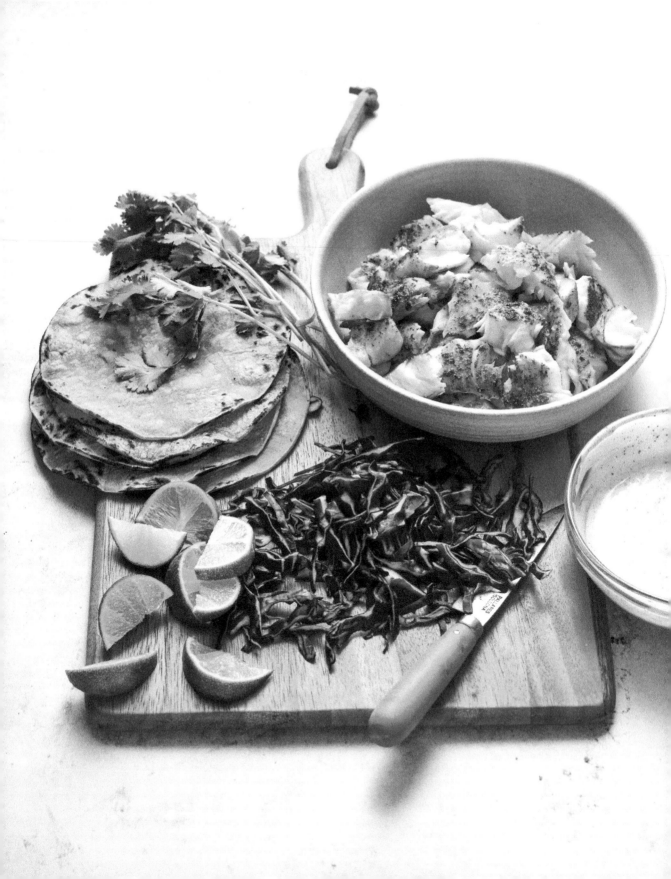

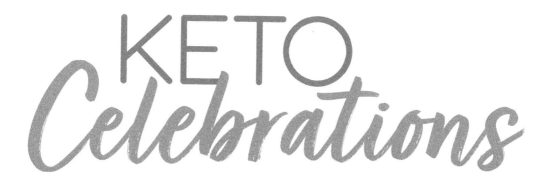

KETO Celebrations

LOW-CARB DISHES FOR HOLIDAYS AND SPECIAL OCCASIONS

MARY ALEXANDER

PHOTOGRAPHY BY ANDREW PURCELL

ROCKRIDGE PRESS

For general information on our other products and services or to obtain technical support, please contact our Customer Care Department within the United States at (866) 744-2665, or outside the United States at (510) 253-0500.

Rockridge Press publishes its books in a variety of electronic and print formats. Some content that appears in print may not be available in electronic books, and vice versa.

Interior and Cover Designer: Mando Daniel

Art Producer: Hannah Dickerson

Editor: Ada Fung

Production Editor: Mia Moran

Photography © 2020 Andrew Purcell. Food styling by Carrie Purcell. Author photo courtesy of Zach Alexander.

ISBN: Print 978-1-64739-016-7 | eBook 978-1-64739-017-4

R0

To my sweet mama, who would have absolutely loved making all the recipes with me for this book!

The many trips down memory lane were lovely, simply lovely. xo

Contents

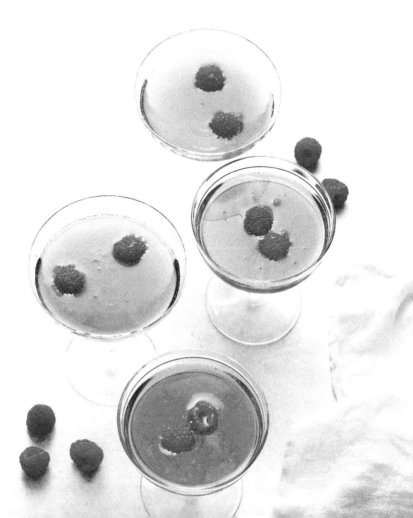

Recipes by Course

Soups and Salads

Broccoli Cheese Soup 123
Cucumber and Tomato Feta Salad 81
Grilled Chicken Cobb Salad 174
Egg Drop Soup 155
Jalapeño Ranch Creamy Coleslaw 73
Matzo Ball Chicken Soup 36
Red Radish "Potato" Salad 80
Strawberry Spinach Salad 164

Sides

Apple Walnut and Pecan Charoset 39
Apricot Cauli-Rice Pilaf 177
Cheesy Mashed Cauliflower 112
Cheesy Mashed Spaghetti Squash 62
Cinnamon Noodle Kugel 91
"Cornbread" Sausage Dressing 110
Cranberry Sauce 113
Creamed Spinach 126
Garlic Breadsticks 165
Garlic Parmesan Asparagus 163
Green Bean Casserole 109
Grilled Avocados 72
Latkes with Sour Cream 127
Oven-Roasted Garlic Green Beans 64
Prosciutto-Wrapped Asparagus and Lemon Aioli 172
Roasted Brussels Slaw 29
Roasted Fall Vegetables 90
Whole Roasted Cauliflower 38

Fish and Seafood

Crab Cakes and Sriracha Mayo 122
Fish Tacos with Chipotle Mayo 51
Garlic Parmesan Crusted Salmon 31
Ginger Scallion Steamed Fish 152
Salmon in Cream Sauce 162

Poultry and Meat

Bacon and Egg Cheeseburgers 70
Bacon Barbecued Chicken 69
Beef and Broccoli Stir-Fry Zoodles 158
Beef Bourguignon Stew 175
Chicken-Fried Steak and Gravy 60
Chicken Potstickers 156
Chicken Quesadillas 195
Chicken Tamale Pie 103
Classic Prime Rib Au Jus 124
Fried Chicken 78
Honey Glazed Ham 28
Roasted Herb Chicken 37
Roast Turkey 108
Slow Cooker Brisket 89
Slow Cooker White Chicken Chili 187
Smoked Ribs 68
Spicy Kung Pao Chicken 154
Thanksgiving Leftovers Pizza 116

Dessert and Sweet Treats

Almond Cookies 159
Apple Pie Bites 74
Baked Donut Bites with Jelly 129
Butter Cake with Cream Cheese Buttercream 178
Chocolate Fudge 167
Chocolate Marble Pound Cake 148
Chocolate Whoopie Pies 188
Churros and Chocolate Sauce 54
Cobweb Brownies 96
Pan de Muertos 102

Drinks

Introduction

When I started keto on Valentine's Day 2016, it was on the heels of many diet debacles. I had spent a good 30 years of my life doing what I call "yo-yo dieting." The idea of eating normally and sensibly didn't work for me. I was a binger, and every diet I tried resulted in a few pounds lost followed by a gain of even more because I would reward myself with food. Lose a pound? Time for a cookie! At 52 years old and 60-plus pounds overweight, I knew I had to do something fast, not just to regain my self-esteem but to save my life.

When I discovered keto, it filled my need for satisfying food. The wide variety of delicious high-fat foods along with adequate amounts of protein kept me satisfied and full. The absence of carbs stopped the sugar roller coaster that kept me binging and craving sweets, and suddenly, I was doing it. I was losing weight, I was mindful of what I was eating, and I was content!

However, I did miss one thing: I couldn't imagine not having all the holiday food that I grew up with and missing the family and love that surrounded it, so I decided to use holiday food as a reward. During my first year on keto, I set up celebration "cheat" days for special occasions. I would buckle down and make it to those days and then totally twist off, eat everything in sight, and gain back much of what I had worked so hard to lose.

I came home from a trip to Mexico to find I had gained 12 pounds—that's when all the cheating stopped. I decided to celebrate with foods that were keto-friendly instead of celebrating with foods that weren't, and that's when the magic happened. I was finally in control, and keto became more than a diet—it became a lifestyle that I knew I could live with.

I owned a specialty cake business for years, so I understand the connection between celebration and food. But my experience here also meant that I could use my baking and recipe development talents to come up with dishes that were keto-friendly *and* holiday-friendly. I began to take our favorite pre-keto foods and swap out ingredients for keto-friendly choices to the delight of my family and to the surprise of others who had no idea they weren't eating traditional carb-laden versions.

I know so many of you are in the same boat. Keto is such a wonderful lifestyle, but it's also hard to miss out on the favorite foods you grew up with and love, especially when special occasions roll around. That's why I wrote this book. Now you can have your celebratory food and feel good about it! You can savor holiday meals just like you remember doing and still maintain your keto way of life.

HOW TO USE THIS BOOK

The recipes in this book are balanced between sweet and savory dishes and organized by season. Each chapter is broken down into different holidays or occasions, each of which includes three to six recipes to make up a well-rounded menu. I've even included a chapter on keto-friendly cocktails that you can mix and match and pair with any occasion. I'm hoping these recipes will become favorites you can enjoy on special occasions, but many of them are also dishes that would be at home on your dinner table any day of the week. That's why I've also included an alternate table of contents, with the recipes organized by course, so you can more easily find the recipe you're looking for.

Each recipe lists the number of servings for the dish, prep and cooking times, and macros for one serving plus calories, fat, carbohydrates, fiber, protein, sugar alcohols, and net carbs. You may decide you're able to have a larger portion based on the macros, or maybe one that's smaller fits better. Dietary labels will indicate whether a dish is vegetarian, vegan, nut-free, and/or dairy-free to meet any special dietary needs.

I've also included tips for prep, cooking, and customization, such as ways to spice up a recipe or suggestions for other recipes in the book that will pair with it nicely. Happy cooking and celebrating!

Butter Cake with Cream Cheese Buttercream, page 178

PART ONE

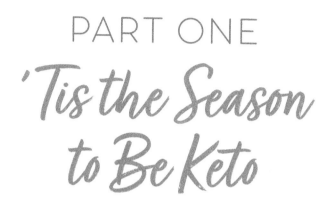

'Tis the Season to Be Keto

Yes, you can have your cake and be keto, too! Before we get to all the fun holiday menus and delicious recipes, let's walk through the basics of the ketogenic diet. We'll explore how to fit holiday food into your keto lifestyle, and I'll share tips on hosting get-togethers and eating out. We'll also cover all the ingredients and cooking equipment you'll need to make and share these wonderful meals with your loved ones.

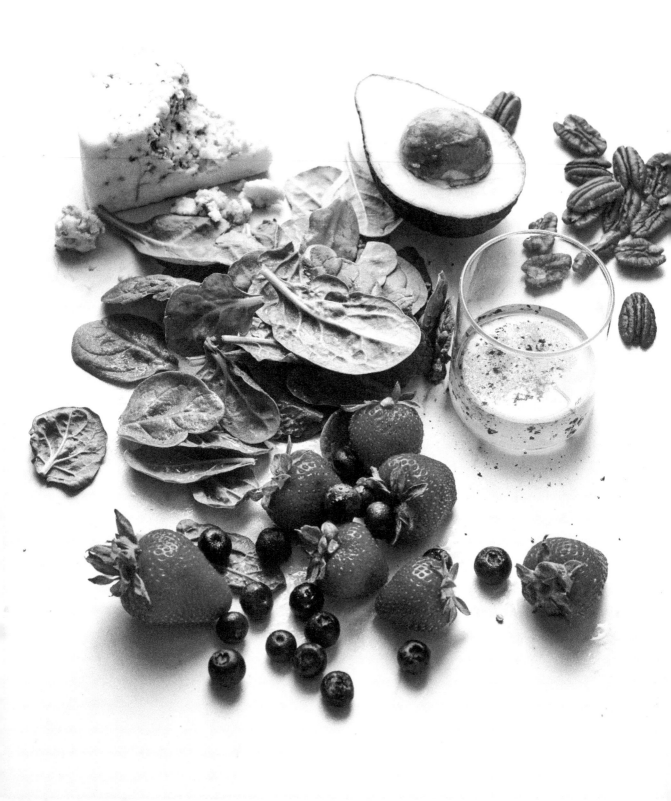

weight loss, but ketones are also considered to be a better source of energy for your brain, which is why so many people on keto report feeling sharper and more energized than those following a traditional diet.

How do we get into ketosis? By eating a low-carb, moderate-protein, and high-fat diet. This way of eating starves our body of its source of glucose (carbs) and supplies it instead with energy from high-quality fats like fatty meats and fish, eggs, nuts, seeds, olive oil, cream, and butter.

You might have heard keto-ers talk about "tracking their macros," or figuring out their macro ratio. Macros, or macronutrients, are the three main building blocks of our food: fat, protein, and carbohydrates. The standard macro ratio for the keto diet is 70 to 75 percent fat, 20 to 25 percent protein, and 5 to 10 percent carbohydrates, meaning that 70 to 75 percent of your calories should come from fat, 20 to 25 percent from protein, and only 5 to 10 percent from carbs.

Not everyone's ideal macro ratios are the same, because everyone's body and health goals are different. If you're very active, you may find that you can maintain ketosis eating a higher percentage of carbohydrates. Free online macro calculators can help you calculate your optimal macros. As you continue your diet, go back and recalculate your macros to fit your progress. I've listed some sites for macro calculators in the Resources section (page 210).

Getting into Ketosis and Staying There

The fastest way to get into ketosis is by restricting your carbohydrates. A good rule of thumb is to stay under 20 net carbs per day. Before you reach ketosis and start burning fat, your body has to burn through all of its glucose and glycogen first, and this can take 2 to 4 days or sometimes longer.

Some signs that you're in ketosis may include weight loss, lack of appetite, and a funky, fruity taste in your mouth or bad breath in general. You may also experience the "keto flu." These flu-like symptoms are caused by the loss of electrolytes and water weight and can make you feel nauseated, run-down, or even sick. You can push past these symptoms by replacing those lost electrolytes with supplements, more water, pickle juice, or warm bone broth.

The trick to staying in ketosis is keeping your carbs low and your fat intake high, tracking your macros, and perhaps testing your ketones using urine strips or the more accurate blood-ketone meter.

KETO-FY YOUR FAMILY FAVORITES

This book includes many traditional holiday dishes, but obviously, your family favorites may not be represented. That doesn't mean they're off-limits. Hopefully, my recipes will serve as inspiration for how you might "keto-fy" your own family's recipes.

Here are some easy swaps to get you started on keto-fying your recipes:

Sugar. My favorite sugar substitutes are ones that you can swap in a 1:1 ratio, like erythritol blends such as Lakanto and Swerve. Stevia is another option, but it's much sweeter than regular sugar.

Flour. For baked goods, almond flour is the closest swap when it comes to measuring 1:1 with traditional flour. Coconut flour is a much thirstier flour, so use ¼ to ⅓ cup of coconut flour to 1 cup of regular flour and add more liquid. I'll typically double the number of eggs and add additional sugar-free almond milk or coconut milk.

Bread crumbs. For breading meats and vegetables, the best swaps are crushed pork skins, almond flour, and grated Parmesan. You could also try flaxseed meal and finely chopped nuts.

Potatoes, rice, and pasta. Cauliflower can be turned into cauliflower rice or boiled or roasted and then mashed for mashed "potatoes." For chunks of potato, try using radishes or turnips, cooked the same way. My favorite swaps for pasta? Spaghetti squash and zucchini noodles, or "zoodles"—both are great for absorbing sauces and flavor.

Apples. Jicama is my favorite hack for mimicking apples in desserts. They have great crunch, too, so you can snack on them raw.

Now go forth and tinker with your family favorites to make them keto! Use a free online net carb/macros recipe calculator (see the Resources section on page 210) to input your ingredients and make sure the end result has keto-friendly macros.

Fitting Holiday Food into Your Keto Life

Of course, the menus and recipes you'll find in this book are all keto-friendly. This means they're sugar-free and lower in carbs than many traditional holiday foods. However, some recipes, especially the baked goods, might be on the higher end of the carb counts that you are aiming for in an ordinary day. Depending on your goals, you can use the nutrition information following each recipe to make choices on how much of that dish you want to spend your daily macros on. For example, if you're planning on having only one big meal, you might go all in. Or maybe you decide on smaller servings of the main dish and splurge on dessert. It's all up to you!

I've also included some fun cocktail recipes to replace some of your sugary favorites. Other good alcoholic drink choices are low-carb beers or a glass of dry white or red wine, which comes in at around 2 carbs. And a flute of champagne has only 1 carb! Liquor such as vodka, whiskey, tequila, and others are typically zero carbs and are great with sugar-free mixers or over ice. My favorite keto-friendly cocktails are Tito's vodka and soda or Jack Daniels and Diet Coke. One thing to remember is that your body burns through alcohol before anything else, so while it might not kick you out of ketosis, it could slow down weight loss. Also, it's important to be cautious about how much you're drinking. Without carbs, alcohol can affect you very quickly.

KEEPIN' IT KETO WHILE DINING OUT

At first, it may seem challenging to stay keto through social events and dining out, but it's actually pretty easy if you know what to do. If you're going to a social event at a restaurant, go online beforehand and peruse the menu. It's a lot easier to make good choices from your laptop than it is in the midst of others ordering up high-carb appetizers, meals, and desserts.

Many appetizers are not keto-friendly, so sometimes it's easier to skip them and move right along to the main meal. Look for meat, poultry, and fish dishes, and ask for any sauces to be put on the side or left off entirely. Ask for roasted or steamed veggies in place of pasta or rice. Many restaurants will offer keto-friendly sides like Brussels sprouts, green beans, spaghetti squash, and others. Don't be afraid to ask how a dish is prepared or ask for substitutions or special preparation. Most restaurants are more than happy to accommodate your requests.

Consider choices like loaded hamburgers or chicken sandwiches served as a salad instead of with bread. Mexican food, such as fajitas minus the tortillas or a salad with lettuce, meat, shredded cheese, and guacamole, is another terrific option. I prefer to ask for sour cream instead of salad dressings, since restaurants will sometimes doctor these up with sugar for taste.

Top Tips for Keto Holiday Success

The holidays are a wonderful time for friends and family to get together, but they can also be stressful. Here are some foolproof and straightforward ways to have fun, stay on track, and navigate special occasions with grace and no feelings of self-deprivation.

Offer to host. This way, you plan the menu and control the majority of what's being served. You can ask folks to bring a side or dessert that they enjoy or assign a few dishes that are popular but not keto-friendly so you don't have to worry about preparing them.

Call ahead and get the scoop. If you aren't in charge of hosting, call ahead and ask what's on the menu and suggest what you'd like to bring. This way, even if you just bring an appetizer or side, you'll be set with something you know is on your plan.

Prep in advance. If you're hosting, prepare foods ahead of time. Many times, I've spent the majority of the party cooking and then not being able to enjoy my guests. Most of the appetizers and dishes in this book can be made ahead, put out minutes before your guests arrive, and then simply replenished or reheated and served.

Go with a full belly. You may not always have the opportunity to host or even take a dish. In these situations, I'll eat ahead of time. If I get to the event and find a charcuterie tray or some other keto-friendly goodies, I'm happily surprised and indulge. If there's nothing that fits my lifestyle, I'm not hungry or as tempted to eat off plan and can still enjoy the party.

Focus on the folks. Ultimately, celebrations are really about quality time with family and friends. Try not to stress over the high-carb sugary foods you can't have and get excited about the foods you can. Use this book and try some fun new dishes or get ideas on how to keto-fy family favorites that comfort you during these special times.

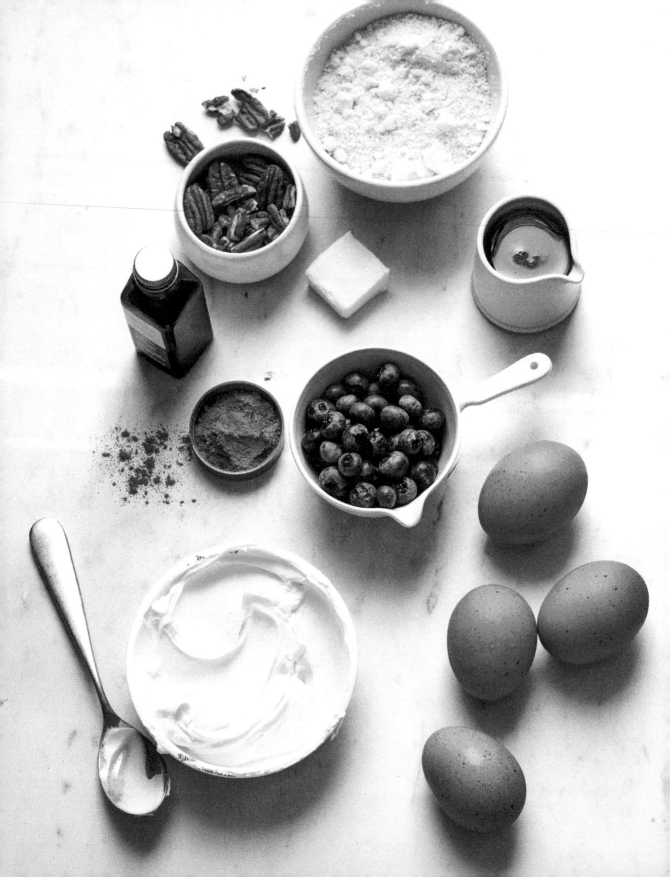

CHAPTER TWO

Your Keto Holiday Kitchen

In this chapter, we'll explore the ingredients and tools used in this book along with some of my favorites that are simply great to have. The good news is that a lot of these items are already in your kitchen!

Keto Pantry Staples

Stocking your pantry ahead of time will make it super easy and convenient when you're ready to try out new recipes or experiment on something new.

Oils and Condiments

Avocado oil. This is my favorite oil for baking, and I prefer the refined version (less avocado-y taste). Because it has a medium to high smoke point, I also use it a lot for sautéing and panfrying. Primal Kitchen is my favorite brand, although I also enjoy trying new varieties that I find on my travels.

Coconut oil, lard, and tallow. I like these for cooking and baking.

Nuts and nut butter. These are popular items at our house. Pecans are the most keto-friendly, but we also love macadamia nuts and almonds. Nut butters are great for snacking or for using in baked or savory dishes. Justin's Nut Butter has a multitude of flavors in packets and jars and is available just about everywhere.

Olive oil. I don't know what I would do without olive oil in my house! I use regular for everything except dips, in which I use extra-virgin.

Peanut oil. When it comes to deep-frying, I like to use peanut oil. It's not the best choice when it comes to keto, but I don't deep-fry often enough to recycle the oil, so it's the least expensive "good keto choice" for me based on volume needed and ease.

Vinegar. I keep apple cider, balsamic, and white vinegars on hand. These are all great for flavoring recipes and homemade sauces.

Canned, Jarred, and Dried Goods

Bone broth. Kettle & Fire is the brand we love and use just about daily for soup and recipes or just warmed up to drink as a snack.

Canned and jarred vegetables. Some of the canned and jarred vegetables I love to use in recipes are olives, green chiles, roasted red peppers, and crushed tomatoes.

Canned chicken and tinned fish. I love canned chicken or tuna to make salads or canned salmon for salmon patties.

Canned pumpkin. Another great ingredient for baked or savory dishes.

Coconut cream. I love this for baked and savory dishes.

Dried or fresh herbs. If you buy fresh herbs, their flavor is the best when crushed between your fingers or ground in a mortar and pestle. Fresh or dried herbs can be sautéed in oil before use to wake up the aroma and flavor.

Pork skins. Great for snacking, these come packaged like chips or crushed for breading. I like to add them on top of a casserole for a little extra crunch.

Spices and seasonings. These are my secret weapon. Most are keto-friendly, so stock up on garlic powder, cumin, cayenne, and Lawry's seasoned salt, along with all your other favorites. Some others I like are cream of tartar, pumpkin and apple pie spice, cinnamon, and nutmeg. Some packaged mixes can be keto-friendly in small doses, like taco seasoning and ranch dressing mix. I also include soy sauce, sesame seed oil, and red pepper flakes in many recipes.

Countertop Items

We've all been in the middle of fixing dinner only to find there's no onion. For that reason, I buy a small red onion and white onion almost every time I visit the market. Some others to add to the "countertop list" are avocados, peppers, garlic, tomatoes, eggplant, ginger, lemons, limes, jicama (to sub for apples), spaghetti squash, and zucchini.

Refrigerated and Frozen Keto Essentials

Here, I'll share the refrigerated and frozen staples that my kitchen is never without because I find them key to keto success.

Dairy and Eggs

Butter. I use unsalted butter every day in many of my recipes. Melted, it mixes easily with other ingredients; cold, it can help create pockets of air in baking to crisp things up or make them airy. It's great for flavor and sautéing but not for frying. With its low smoke point, it can quickly burn your dish. My favorite brand is unsalted Kerrygold, which can be found just about anywhere.

Creams. I use sour cream, cream cheese, mascarpone, and heavy whipping cream daily. Steer clear of flavored cream cheeses though, as they tend to have added sugar. Mascarpone, an Italian cream cheese, can be used in many of the same ways as regular cream cheese. Heavy whipping cream is great for baking, puddings, and whipped cream.

Eggs. I like organic brown eggs and usually have at least two dozen in the refrigerator.

Hard cheeses. Mozzarella, Parmesan, and cheddar are our favorites. We use them in recipes and to top salads or pizzas, cheese waffles (aka "chaffles"), and so much more. Cheese is something I'll spend extra money on for a special occasion. I might splurge on a Gruyère for a particular recipe or a Jersey Blue and a white Stilton for a holiday charcuterie tray.

Milks. The nut milks I use in recipes or just to drink are Califia Farms unsweetened vanilla almond milk and Milkadamia unsweetened vanilla milk, but any unsweeetened nut milk of your choice will work in these recipes.

Meats and Seafood

Meats. My partner, Lovies, is an expert when it comes to grilling and smoking food, so we always have an abundance of meat. He'll smoke a big brisket, and we'll eat it for days. Other meats we love to grill are chicken and ribs.

Seafood. I enjoy using salmon in recipes, along with tilapia, cod, and red snapper. Baked, roasted, or fried, they're all delicious! My boys love shrimp, so I'll use it in recipes instead of chicken.

Smoked and cured meats. Bacon and sausage are staples in my fridge. We also enjoy cured meats like meat sticks, jerky, summer sausage, prosciutto, and pepperoni.

A CHARCUTERIE BOARD FIT FOR A PARTY

Charcuterie boards are so much fun to put together and, really, anything goes. I like to include:

- **Meats:** Cured or smoked options like ham, prosciutto, cured sausages, or salami

- **Cheeses:** A variety of cheeses, soft and hard, mellow and strong, like Brie, Gouda, blue cheese, white cheddar, Stiltons, and aged cheddar

- **Veggies:** Sliced cucumber, zucchini, celery sticks, and cherry tomatoes

- **Nuts:** Pecans, almonds, and cashews

- **Berries:** A colorful variety of blueberries, raspberries, blackberries, and strawberries

- **Pickled items:** Mini dill pickles and olives (black, green, stuffed)

- **Condiments:** Little bowls of sugar-free jelly, mustards, and any of the dips in this book (like on pages 94 and 194)

- **Crackers:** Use the cracker or "scoops" recipe on page 136.

For assembly, use a tray, a cutting board, or whatever flat serving platter you have. You want the board to look full, so don't be afraid to pile and stack items with an eye toward color and textures!

Produce

Here's a short list of some of the really good produce for keto—great for roasting, dipping, salads, sauces, and snacking:

- Asparagus
- Berries
- Broccoli
- Brussels sprouts
- Cabbage
- Cauliflower

- Cucumbers
- Jalapeños
- Leafy greens
- Peppers
- Radishes
- Tomatoes

Keto Baking Ingredients

Keto baking is dependent on a variety of swaps, and I've done my homework to make sure baked goods can still be a part of my days, especially holidays. I'm happy to share those products and tips with you.

Keto-Friendly Flours and Meals

Low-carb alternatives for flour are the most challenging ingredients to swap because nothing works quite the way flour does. Each has a unique way of replacing flour, and the more recipes you try, the easier it becomes to use them:

Almond flour. This is the closest 1:1 swap for flour. I use it mostly for crusts, crackers, bars, and breading, where you want a little crunch. My favorite is Bob's Red Mill Super-Fine.

Coconut flour. This works best for cake-like items, making them soft and moist. It's my go-to for pancakes, cookies, cake, and muffins. It's lower in carbs than almond flour because you use less. My favorite is the readily available Bob's Red Mill Organic.

Flaxseed meal. Great for texture in muffins and "cornbread," flaxseed adds a hearty, nutty flavor along with moisture. Golden and brown flaxseed are very much the same, except that the golden version is more aesthetically pleasing. My favorite is Bob's Red Mill Organic Golden Flaxseed Meal.

Whey protein isolate. I like this for pan- and deep-frying. It makes the crispiest breading and is entirely gluten-free, nut-free, grain-free, and pork-free. My favorite brand is Isopure.

Sweeteners

In this book, I mainly use erythritol blends that are a 1:1 swap for sugar. I recommend that you keep these on hand, especially if you plan on doing a lot of holiday baking and cooking:

A brown erythritol blend. I find that Swerve Brown best mimics brown sugar.

A granulated erythritol blend. This is a 1:1 swap for granulated sugar. I like both the monk fruit–erythritol blend from Lakanto and an erythritol-oligosaccharides blend like Swerve. All my recipes call for just a granulated erythritol blend, so you can choose which one you like.

A powdered, or confectioners', erythritol blend. This is a replacement for powdered/confectioners' sugar. Both Lakanto and Swerve have powdered sweeteners.

Coffee and drink sweetener. Liquid Stevia is an excellent keto choice for coffee and drinks.

As a note, I've also used xylitol, which swaps 1:1 with sugar and is good, but it's lethal for pets, so I don't keep it in my house.

Leavening Agents, Thickeners, and Binders

Texture is as important as taste. Here are some good swaps for helping foods rise, thicken, and bind as necessary to achieve the right texture:

Binders. Traditional binders include crackers, bread crumbs, and flour, and I replace these ingredients with crushed pork skins, whey protein isolate, and almond and coconut flour.

Leavening agents. In the keto kitchen, nut flours need a little encouragement to rise, so I use baking soda and baking powder along with buttermilk, which has the acidity to create the necessary rise. You can also beat egg whites separately and fold them in for more lightness.

Thickening agents. I use psyllium husk powder and xanthan gum in soups, sauces, and baked goods.

Flavoring Agents and Extras

Extracts are probably the easiest way to add sweet and fruity flavors to foods. You can find many flavors alongside the vanilla in the baking section of your market, but my favorites to use are LorAnn Oils. Sold in hobby and craft stores, they're much stronger than traditional extracts and come in a multitude of flavors. Other ingredients I regularly use for flavor are Hershey's unsweetened cocoa powder, sugar-free jams and jellies, Lily's sugar-free chocolate chips, and unsweetened shredded coconut. There are many other options, but just be sure to read the labels and check for carbs as you experiment.

Your Keto Holiday Kitchen Equipment

No expensive or specialized equipment is needed to make great foods on the keto diet; in fact, if you cook or bake, you're probably already most of the way there. We'll walk through the essentials and some extras that are nice to have.

The Essentials

Baking pans. A good variety to have includes:

- Large metal baking sheet for roasting vegetables, cookies, biscuits, and more

- Standard 12-cup muffin pan and mini muffin pan

- 9-by-13-inch baking pan with straight sides for brownies and bars

- Loaf pan

- 2 (7- or 8-inch) round pans with straight sides, as well as an 8- or 9-inch glass pie pan

Cookie scoop. This tool is great for measuring equal amounts of anything that will be rolled into a ball.

Knives. The three I use the most are a chef's knife for chopping, serrated knife for slicing, and small paring knife for peeling.

Measuring tools. Measuring spoons and cups for dry and liquid ingredients are at the top of the list. An inexpensive food scale is also invaluable for measuring ingredients in ounces.

Metal cooling racks. Perfect for cooling foods right out of the oven and also useful for setting in pans for roasting chicken and more.

Mixing bowls. You'll want at least one or two medium to large bowls and smaller ones as well. Plastic, metal, and glass are all great.

Mixing tools. Rubber and silicone spatulas, a whisk, and an electric hand mixer will get used often.

Parchment paper, foil, and muffin tin liners. Parchment paper is great for lining pans for less mess or for rolling out dough. Paper liners for muffins and heavy-duty aluminum foil are great to have as well.

Piping bags and tips. Plan on entertaining? Get some piping bags and tips— they're pretty inexpensive, usually under $10. They're so perfect for making holiday food look fancy and will also come in handy for everyday meals. My favorite tip is the larger star tip, Ateco #824 or Wilton's 1M.

Pots and pans. I recommend having a few frying pans and pots in a variety of sizes. (All-Clad is my favorite brand.) I also suggest getting a heavy-bottomed 4-quart stockpot if you don't already have one.

Blender. Perfect for mixing smoothies, drinks, and sauces.

Candy thermometer. Good for keeping oil at the correct temperature when deep-frying.

Silicone cupcake pan and donut pan. I love that you don't need to grease these—and your baked goods pop out perfectly every time! Silicone is also great for candy molds, which are fun to collect in different holiday themes.

Slow cooker. It's so rewarding to throw in a roast, let it cook and tenderize all day long, and have dinner waiting when you get home.

Spiral slicer. This tool, also called a spiralizer, makes noodles out of vegetables like zucchini (called "zoodles"). You'll find many uses for it.

Techniques for Holiday Keto Foods

In chapter 1, I gave you some simple keto-approved swaps for popular ingredients in holiday foods. Here, I offer up some of my tried-and-tested tips for working with keto ingredients you might not be super familiar with.

Comfort Carbs

Here are some ways to prep and cook my favorite keto-friendly carb swaps:

Cauliflower. Cut cauliflower into florets, coat with olive oil, spread on parchment paper, and roast in a 425°F oven for 30 to 45 minutes. Then chop up the florets and use as rice or puree for imitation mashed potatoes. This method also works for turnips and radishes.

Spaghetti squash. Another great pasta swap. Just cut the squash in half, remove seeds, lay facedown on parchment paper, roast at 425°F for 30 to 45 minutes until fork-tender, and then use a fork to scrape out all the spaghetti squash for noodles.

Zoodles (zucchini noodles). These make a wonderful stand-in for pasta. You can use a grater, but a spiralizer is the easiest way to make noodles from zucchini or squash.

Crunchy Fried Foods

Here are a few hacks to ensure perfectly crunchy results:

Enlist keto breadings. Products like almond flour and pork rinds make wonderful breadings. Whey protein isolate is great for foods like fried chicken. Just coat the item in a buttermilk and egg mixture and then in the breading mixture, and drop it right into the hot oil.

Test the oil. A candy thermometer will tell you when you've reached the right temperature (350 to 375°F). Alternately, use the wooden spoon method. When you dip a wooden spoon in the oil and bubbles form around the spoon, it's hot enough for frying. If no bubbles form, it's not there yet, and if it bubbles vigorously, it's too hot.

Baked Goods and Desserts

Here are some tips for working with keto ingredients in baking:

Add eggs methodically. To make baked goods lighter, mix the yolks in with the flour and dry ingredients, and then whip the whites separately and fold them in with the batter at the end.

Adjust the temperature. If you find your baked goods are browning too quickly, turn your oven down 20 or 25 degrees and cover your dish with foil.

Consider structure and texture. Keto baking recipes tend to need more eggs and extra baking powder or baking soda to help with structure and rise. This is easy when you follow my recipes but can become an issue when you start experimenting on your own!

Cool thoroughly. Keto baked goods can be a little crumblier than traditional ones, so cooling will help them better hold their shape when you handle them.

Use wet hands. Keto doughs can be a little stickier than regular doughs. Keep your hands and/or spatula a little wet so the dough doesn't stick as you work with it.

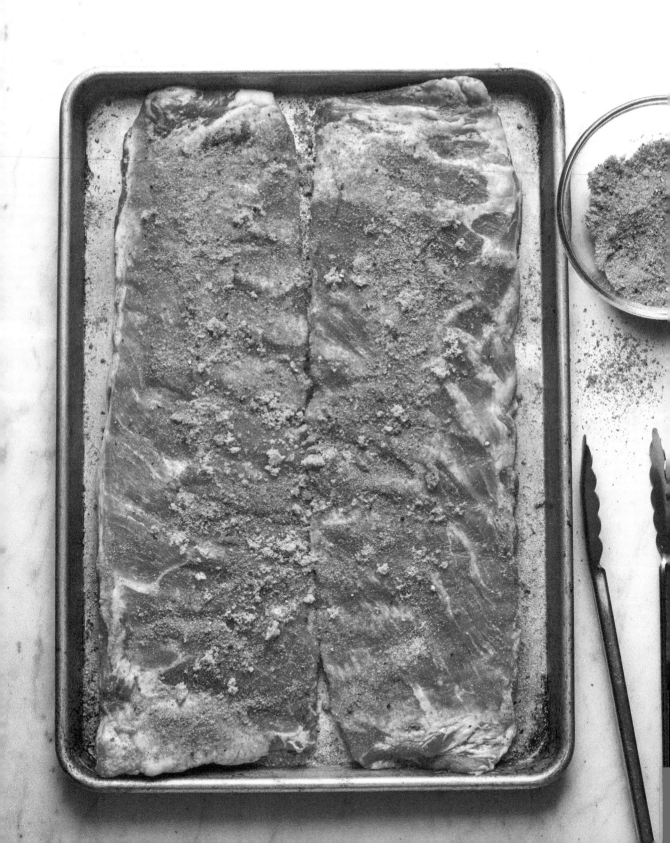

PART TWO

Recipes to Celebrate All Year Round

Now we get to the fun part! Here you'll find all the recipes you need to celebrate—and stay keto—all year round. Chapters are organized by seasons and include menus for some of the most popular holidays of each season. There's also an "anytime" chapter and a bonus cocktails chapter for spirited fun! You might celebrate some of these occasions already, while others may not be part of your family's tradition. Either way, these chapters are full of delicious comfort foods you can prepare and enjoy any day of the year.

CHAPTER THREE

Spring Soirees

Spring is all about new life! Whether your ode to the season is the joyfulness of spring holidays or just the smell of freshly cut grass, I've got you covered with the season's best from my celebratory recipe files. Get in the spirit with traditional Easter favorites, a beautiful Passover dinner, and a well-deserved Mother's Day Breakfast in Bed, and then spice things up with a Cinco de Mayo Fiesta!

Easter Brunch

Honey Glazed Ham (page 28)
Roasted Brussels Slaw (page 29)
Southern Fried Deviled Eggs (page 30)
Garlic Parmesan Crusted Salmon (page 31)
Apricot Hot Cross Buns (page 32)

Southern Fried Deviled Eggs, page 30

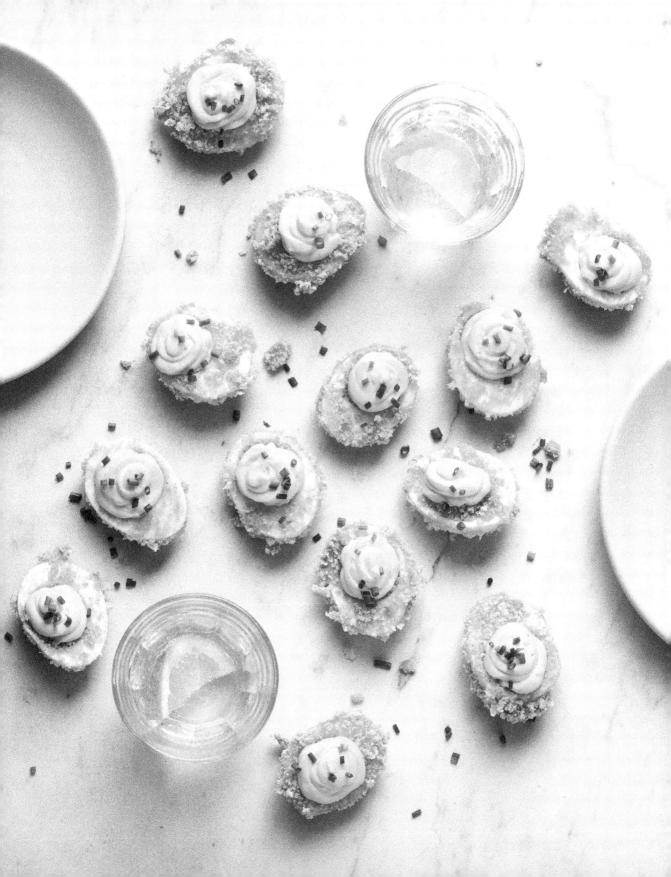

Honey Glazed Ham

NUT-FREE

Prep time: 15 minutes | **Cook time:** 1 hour 30 minutes | **Servings:** 8

Nothing says Easter more than a honey glazed ham. The sticky glaze on the salty ham is just dreamy, and I can't even begin to tell you how many hours I've spent standing in line at the Honey Baked Ham store waiting on its greatness. I had no idea just how simple this recipe could be until I keto-fied it! You'll want to plan on three-quarters of a pound per person. If you want leftovers, go bigger!

1 cup water

4- to 6-pound fully cooked spiral bone-in ham, room temperature, patted dry

½ cup brown erythritol blend

½ cup sugar-free apricot preserves

2 tablespoons butter, room temperature

1. Preheat the oven to 300°F and line a large roasting pan with heavy aluminum foil.

2. Pour 1 cup of water into the pan, and lay the ham on its side in the pan.

3. In a small bowl, mix the brown sweetener, apricot preserves, and butter into a paste. Rub half of the paste over the ham, especially in between the spiral cuts.

4. Cover gently with foil, and bake for 1 hour.

5. Carefully remove the ham from the oven. Spoon out about ¼ cup of juice from the bottom of the pan and mix it with the remaining brown sugar paste. Using half of the mixture, baste the ham and place back in the oven, uncovered, for another 25 minutes.

6. Carefully remove the ham from the oven and increase the temperature to broil. Baste the ham with the remaining mixture, return to the oven, and broil for 3 to 5 minutes, watching so it doesn't burn.

7. Remove from the oven and let sit for at least 15 to 20 minutes before serving.

Per Serving: Calories: 239; Total Fat: 10g; Carbohydrates: 11g; Fiber: 2g; Net Carbs: 3g; Protein: 33g; Sugar Alcohols: 6g
Macros: Fat 38% Carbs 5% Protein 55%

Roasted Brussels Slaw

NUT-FREE, VEGETARIAN

Prep time: 15 minutes | **Cook time:** 25 minutes | **Servings:** 8

I love a fancy vegetable at Easter, and there's nothing more elegant than roasted Brussels sprouts. This slaw version will turn even the biggest skeptic into a Brussels sprouts lover. I especially like that it can be prepped in advance and stored in the refrigerator until roasting time, making it an easy addition to a weekly dinner rotation as well. You could also toss in some crispy bacon and use the bacon grease instead of the oil.

24 ounces Brussels sprouts

4 tablespoons olive oil or avocado oil

1 teaspoon garlic salt

1 teaspoon freshly ground black pepper

¼ cup finely grated Parmesan cheese

1. Preheat the oven to 400°F, and line a baking dish with parchment paper. Set aside.
2. Cut the ends off the Brussels sprouts, peel off and discard any wilted leaves, and thinly slice the sprouts.
3. Place the Brussels sprouts into a gallon resealable bag and add the oil. Seal, and gently massage and turn the bag until the slices are coated.
4. Spread the slices evenly on the lined baking sheet. Sprinkle the Brussels sprouts with the garlic salt and pepper.
5. Bake for 20 to 25 minutes, or until the edges are golden but not burned.
6. Remove from the oven, place in a serving dish, and sprinkle with the Parmesan cheese.

PREP TIP

I enjoy hand-slicing the Brussels sprouts, but a food processor is faster. Just be careful not to process them too much or you'll have mush.

Per Serving: Calories: 107; Total Fat: 7.5g; Carbohydrates: 8g; Fiber: 3g; Net Carbs: 5g; Protein: 3g; Sugar Alcohols: 0g
Macros: Fat 63% Carbs 19% Protein 11%

Southern Fried Deviled Eggs

NUT-FREE

Prep time: 15 minutes | **Cook time:** 20 minutes | **Deviled eggs:** 16

Growing up in Texas, we had deviled eggs all the time. When it comes to occasions as special as Easter, we deep-fry them. My favorite oil for deep-frying is avocado oil, but you could also use coconut oil, tallow (beef fat), or lard (pig fat).

4 to 5 cups avocado oil for frying (or enough to fill your pan about 2 inches deep)

8 hard-boiled eggs, plus 2 uncooked eggs

1 cup finely crushed pork skins

¼ cup mayonnaise

¼ cup sour cream

2 teaspoons Dijon mustard

1 teaspoon salt

½ teaspoon freshly ground black pepper

Paprika, for garnish

1. Pour the oil into a deep, medium heavy-bottomed pan, and place on the stove over medium heat.

2. Cut the boiled eggs in half lengthwise. Scoop out the yolks, place the yolks in a small bowl, and set the yolks and egg white boats aside.

3. Pour the crushed pork skins into a shallow bowl. In another shallow bowl, whisk the two uncooked eggs.

4. Take an egg white boat, dip both sides in the pork skins, then submerge it in the whisked eggs and then back in the pork skins. Place on a plate, and repeat with the remaining egg white boats.

5. Using a slotted spoon, gently lower 2 or 3 of the boats into the oil. Cook for about 3 minutes, flipping halfway through, until golden brown. Transfer onto another plate lined with paper towels. Working in batches, repeat with the remaining boats.

6. With a fork, mash the egg yolks. Add the mayonnaise, sour cream, Dijon mustard, salt, and pepper, and mix well. Using a piping bag, resealable bag with the corner cut off, or spoon, fill each boat with yolk mixture, and garnish with paprika.

Per Serving (2 deviled eggs): Calories: 257; Total Fat: 22g; Carbohydrates: 1g; Fiber: 0g; Net Carbs: 1g; Protein: 12g; Sugar Alcohols: 0g
Macros: Fat 77% Carbs 2% Protein 19%

Garlic Parmesan Crusted Salmon

NUT-FREE

Prep time: 15 minutes | **Cook time:** 15 minutes | **Servings:** 8

Garlic Parmesan *anything* sounds good to me, but especially salmon. This recipe is a family favorite that I turn to time and time again. It's great to serve any day of the week but also looks so fancy that it's perfect for special occasions as well. You could also add some asparagus or broccoli on the sides of your baking dish, sprinkle with olive oil or butter, and have a complete meal.

4 pounds salmon
  fillets, skin on
½ cup (1 stick)
  butter, melted
3 cloves garlic, minced

1 teaspoon salt
½ teaspoon freshly ground
  black pepper
½ cup finely crushed
  pork skins

½ cup grated
  Parmesan cheese
1 lemon, for squeezing
  (optional)

1. Preheat the oven to 350°F, and line a baking sheet with parchment paper.
2. Place the salmon fillets, skin-side down, on the lined baking sheet.
3. In a small bowl, mix the butter and minced garlic. Spread or brush over the salmon.
4. Season the fillets with the salt and pepper, and then sprinkle with the crushed pork skins and Parmesan.
5. Bake for 15 minutes, remove from the oven, and squeeze lemon over the top (if using).

COOKING TIP
If you forget to thaw the salmon, you can also cook this dish the same way from frozen. Just increase cooking time by 5 or 10 minutes, checking to make sure it's flaky in the center.

Per Serving: Calories: 532; Total Fat: 32g; Carbohydrates: 1g; Fiber: 0g; Net Carbs: 1g; Protein: 56g; Sugar Alcohols: 0g
Macros: Fat 54% Carbs 1% Protein 42%

Apricot Hot Cross Buns

NUT-FREE, VEGETARIAN

Prep time: 15 minutes | **Cook time:** 15 minutes | **Rolls:** 12

When I was a kid, we always had hot cross buns for Easter. They would hit the shelves of the grocery store, and it would be a frenzied scene of shoppers grabbing them up. As I got older and learned to bake, I decided to take on these sweet buns, and my homemade version turned out even better. Keto-fying them has been a little challenging, but I think I've gotten it down and know you'll enjoy them, too.

FOR THE BUNS

¼ cup (½ stick) melted butter, plus more for greasing

1 cup whey protein isolate, unflavored

½ cup flaxseed meal

½ cup coconut flour

¼ cup granulated erythritol blend

2 teaspoons baking powder

3 large eggs

1 teaspoon xanthan gum

1 tablespoon olive oil

½ cup heavy cream

1 teaspoon cream of tartar

4 tablespoons sugar-free apricot preserves

FOR THE ICING

2 ounces (4 tablespoons) cream cheese, melted slightly in microwave

¼ cup confectioners' erythritol blend

1. Preheat the oven to 350°F, and heavily grease a muffin pan with melted butter.

2. **To make the buns:** In a medium bowl, combine the whey protein, flaxseed, flour, sweetener, and baking powder. Stir with a fork to break up any lumps.

3. Separate the eggs. Add the yolks to the flour mixture, and put the whites in a medium metal bowl.

4. Add the melted butter, olive oil, and cream to the flour mixture, and mix just until incorporated. Don't overmix.

5. Add the cream of tartar to the whites in the metal bowl. Using a mixer, beat the whites until they form small peaks. Gently fold the whites into the flour mixture until just incorporated.

6. Evenly spoon the mixture into the 12 muffin holes, and bake for 10 minutes.

7. **To make the icing:** Mix together the melted cream cheese and confectioners' blend. Add the icing to a piping bag or resealable bag with the corner cut off.

8. When the buns are baked, brush a coat of apricot preserves across the top of each bun. Pipe an icing cross on each one, and bake for another 3 to 5 minutes.

9. Remove from the oven, and let them sit for about 5 minutes before removing from the pan.

SWAP IT

These sweet buns would also be great as rolls without the jam or cross on top. Just brush butter across the top of each one instead.

Per Serving (1 roll): Calories: 233; Total Fat: 14g; Carbohydrates: 14g; Fiber: 4g; Net Carbs: 3.5g; Protein: 21g; Sugar Alcohols: 6.5g
Macros: Fat 54% Carbs 6% Protein 36%

Passover Dinner

Matzo Ball Chicken Soup (page 36)
Roasted Herb Chicken (page 37)
Whole Roasted Cauliflower (page 38)
Apple Walnut and Pecan Charoset (page 39)

Matzo Ball Chicken Soup, page 36

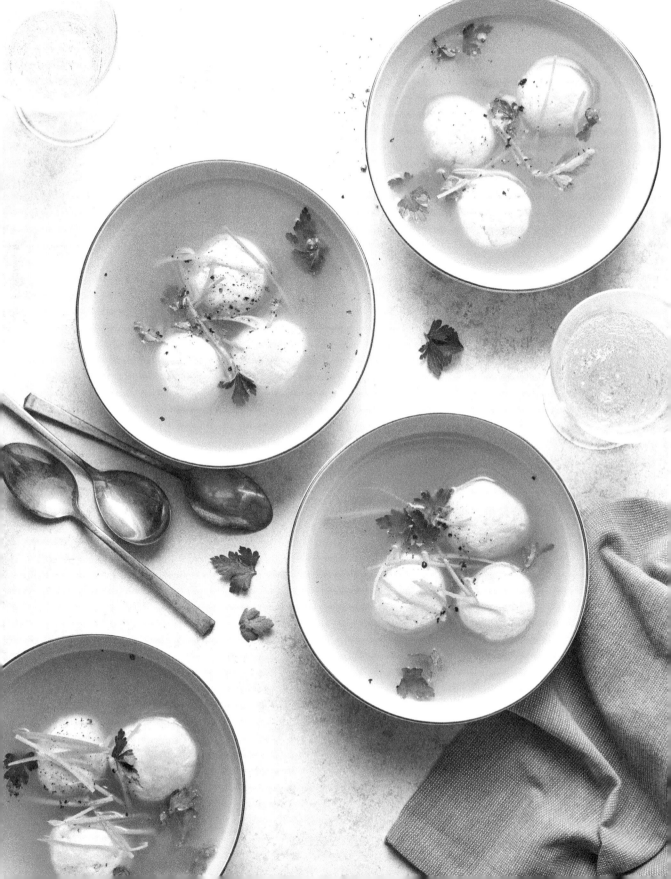

Matzo Ball Chicken Soup

DAIRY-FREE

Prep time: 10 minutes, plus 2 hours to chill | **Cook time:** 30 minutes | **Servings:** 6

Passover just wouldn't be the same without matzo ball soup. Matzo ball dough can be mixed dense to make sinkers or airy to make floaters. The balls can be cooked in water so the chicken soup remains clear or cooked in the chicken broth, making the matzo balls much tastier but the broth a little cloudy. However you like yours, there's nothing more soothing and delicious than a bowl of chicken broth with a matzo ball swimming in it.

3 large eggs

½ teaspoon salt

1 teaspoon freshly ground black pepper

2 cups almond flour

2 tablespoons coconut flour

1 teaspoon baking powder

1 tablespoon olive oil

6 cups chicken bone broth

1 carrot, shredded, for garnish

1. In a small bowl, whisk the eggs, salt, and pepper for 1 minute.

2. In a large bowl, mix together the almond flour, coconut flour, and baking powder. Use a fork to mash out any lumps.

3. Add the egg mixture and oil to the flour mixture, and stir just until incorporated. Cover and place in the refrigerator for 2 hours or up to overnight.

4. After chilling the dough, place a medium stockpot on the stove over medium heat, and pour the bone broth into the pot.

5. Remove the mixture from the refrigerator, and using a cookie scoop, roll a ball the size of a Ping-Pong ball in the palm of your hand. Repeat for a total of 18 matzo balls.

6. When the broth comes to a boil, carefully lower each ball into the pot using a slotted spoon, reduce heat to a simmer, and cook for 30 minutes.

7. Ladle 1 cup of broth and 3 matzo balls into each bowl, and garnish with shredded carrots.

SPICE IT UP

To make this soup more of a meal, add some leftover chicken from the Roasted Herb Chicken (page 37) or any other kind of chicken you'd like.

Per Serving: Calories: 297; Total Fat: 21g; Carbohydrates: 8g; Fiber: 5.5g; Net Carbs: 2.5g; Protein: 19g; Sugar Alcohols: 0g
Macros: Fat 64% Carbs 3% Protein 26%

Roasted Herb Chicken

NUT-FREE

Prep time: 15 minutes | **Cook time:** 1 hour 30 minutes | **Servings:** 6

When I was growing up, my mother's roasted chicken was a favorite of mine. The whole house smelled wonderful as the chicken cooked, and I savored every bite. Once I had my own family, I began roasting chicken, and all the memories flooded back to me from when I was a kid. You can serve this as an elegant showpiece for a special occasion like Passover or any day of the week. The leftovers are also delicious as chicken salad the next day.

½ cup (1 stick) butter, room temperature

2 tablespoons olive oil or avocado oil

3 garlic cloves, minced

1 tablespoon rosemary

1 tablespoon thyme

1 teaspoon garlic salt

1 teaspoon freshly ground black pepper

Juice of ½ lemon

5- to 6-pound whole chicken, room temperature, patted dry, and giblets and neck removed

Chopped parsley, for garnish

1. Preheat the oven to 425°F, and line a roasting pan with aluminum foil.

2. In a small bowl, mix together the butter, oil, garlic, rosemary, thyme, garlic salt, pepper, and lemon juice.

3. Gently loosen the skin on the chicken, and rub the mixture under each area as far as you can reach and all over the outer skin and bottom. Tie the chicken legs together with string.

4. Set a rack in the roasting pan and the chicken, breast-side up, on top of the rack. Roast for 90 minutes, basting every 30 minutes using the juices in the bottom of the pan. If it starts to brown too much toward the end, lay a piece of foil loosely over the top.

5. Remove the pan from the oven, and make a cut between the leg and thigh to test if it's done. If the juices run clear, it's cooked. If there is any pink in the juice, return to the oven and check again in 5 to 10 minutes. Garnish with chopped parsley, and serve.

Per Serving: Calories: 563; Total Fat: 37g; Carbohydrates: 0g; Fiber: 0g; Net Carbs: 0g; Protein: 54g; Sugar Alcohols: 0g
Macros: Fat 59% Carbs 0% Protein 38%

Whole Roasted Cauliflower

NUT-FREE, VEGETARIAN

Prep time: 15 minutes | **Cook time:** 1 hour 10 minutes | **Servings:** 6

I wasn't a fan of cauliflower until I started keto, when a whole new way of roasting vegetables rocked my world. Today, it's one of my favorites. I originally found this dish at a very upscale restaurant served as an appetizer. Ever since, I have prepared it many times to impress. Adding different seasonings can create infinite flavors for any occasion.

1 large cauliflower head, with leaves cut off the bottom

⅓ cup melted butter or olive oil

2 garlic cloves, minced

1 teaspoon salt

½ teaspoon freshly ground black pepper

½ cup grated Parmesan cheese, divided

1 tablespoon chopped parsley, for garnish

1. Preheat the oven to 375°F, and line a small baking dish with aluminum foil.
2. Carefully cut off the bottom of the cauliflower so it sits flat in the pan, being careful not to break off any florets.
3. In a small bowl, mix together the butter, garlic, salt, and pepper. Brush the mixture all over the cauliflower.
4. Cover with foil and bake for 45 minutes; then remove the foil and bake for another 15 minutes, or until fork-tender.
5. Remove from the oven, and increase the heat to broil. Pat about three-quarters of the Parmesan cheese all over the cauliflower. Return to the oven, uncovered, for a few minutes, until the cheese is melted and golden brown.
6. Remove from the oven, sprinkle with the remaining Parmesan, and garnish with the parsley. Stick a knife in the top for presentation, and serve.

SPICE IT UP

This dish is great as a stand-alone vegetable alongside any meal, but when I met it as an appetizer, it was served with a lemon dill yogurt dip. I've paired it since then with ranch and many other keto-friendly dips, and they're all sensational.

Per Serving: Calories: 155; Total Fat: 12g; Carbohydrates: 8.5g; Fiber: 3g; Net Carbs: 5.5g; Protein: 5g; Sugar Alcohols: 0g
Macros: Fat 70% Carbs 14% Protein 13%

Apple Walnut and Pecan Charoset

DAIRY-FREE, VEGAN

Prep time: 15 minutes | **Cook time:** 10 minutes | **Servings:** 6

Charoset is a traditional food eaten as part of the Passover Seder ritual. It represents the mortar the Hebrews used to set bricks while in captivity in Egypt. The main ingredient in many Ashkenazi Jewish recipes is apple, which I have mimicked using jicama. I think a Cabernet Sauvignon is perfect for this dish, but you can use any dry red wine of your choice. I could eat the whole bowl, with or without the wine. It will last in the refrigerator a few days, so if you have leftovers, try some for breakfast over a little Greek yogurt or by itself as a snack. It's that good!

½ cup pecans
½ cup walnuts

2 jicamas, peeled and finely chopped in ¼-inch cubes (about 4 cups chopped)
½ teaspoon cinnamon

1 teaspoon apple pie spice
2 tablespoons brown erythritol blend
⅓ cup Cabernet, or dry red wine of your choice

1. Preheat the oven to 350°F, and line a baking sheet with parchment paper.

2. Spread the pecans and walnuts evenly on the baking sheet, and bake for 8 to 10 minutes, until they have a little color, shaking about halfway through. Allow the nuts to cool, and then coarsely chop them.

3. In a medium bowl, combine the nuts, jicamas, cinnamon, apple pie spice, brown sweetener, and wine, mix well, and serve.

SWAP IT
If you don't have apple pie spice or can't find it in the store, replace it with ½ teaspoon nutmeg, ¼ teaspoon allspice, and an additional ¼ teaspoon of cinnamon.

Per Serving (¾ cup): Calories: 206; Total Fat: 12g; Carbohydrates: 24g; Fiber: 12g; Net Carbs: 10g; Protein: 3g; Sugar Alcohols: 2g
Macros: Fat 52% Carbs 19% Protein 6%

Mother's Day Breakfast in Bed

Ham and Cheese Crustless Quiche (page 42)
Mary's Cinnamon Rolls (page 43)
Raspberry Lemonade (page 45)

Mary's Cinnamon Rolls, page 43

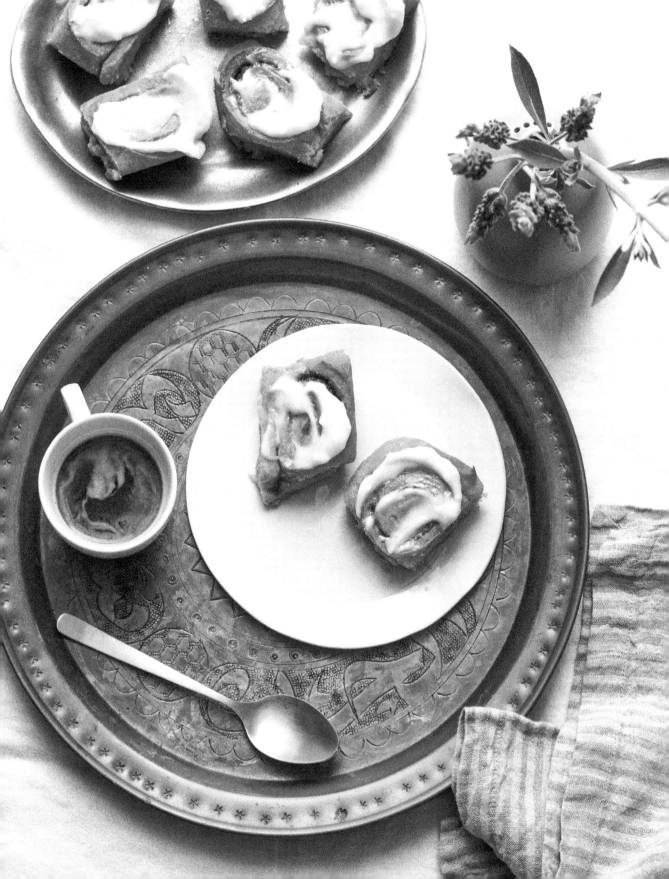

Ham and Cheese Crustless Quiche

NUT-FREE

Prep time: 15 minutes | **Cook time:** 40 minutes | **Servings:** 6

There's no one more worthy of a fancy breakfast in bed than Mom, and being that I'm a mom, my vote is for quiche. It's the prettiest dish to serve, and though there are a million ways to make it, my favorite is crustless ham and cheese. For a little extra flavor, top each serving with some sour cream or hot sauce. Be careful to use a regular cut of ham and not a sugary sweet honey baked or glazed version.

- 1 tablespoon butter or nonstick cooking spray, for greasing
- 1 cup broccoli florets, steamed and chopped
- 6 ounces ham, cut into ¼-inch cubes
- ½ cup grated mozzarella cheese
- ½ cup grated sharp cheddar cheese
- 1 cup heavy cream
- 6 large eggs
- 2 ounces (4 tablespoons) cream cheese
- 1 teaspoon garlic salt
- 1 teaspoon freshly ground black pepper
- 1 teaspoon paprika

1. Preheat the oven to 375°F. Grease a pie pan with butter or cooking spray.
2. Sprinkle the chopped broccoli, ham, mozzarella, and cheddar cheese evenly in the pie pan.
3. Using a hand mixer or blender, mix the cream, eggs, cream cheese, garlic salt, pepper, and paprika until well blended, about 15 seconds. Pour the egg mixture over the ham and broccoli mixture.
4. Bake for 40 to 45 minutes, or until a knife comes out clean when inserted in the middle of the quiche. Remove from the oven and allow to sit for 5 to 10 minutes before slicing and serving.

SWAP IT
The ham can be replaced with any other meat you enjoy. Crispy bacon, cooked sausage, and chorizo are all great substitutions.

Per Serving: Calories: 357; Total Fat: 30g; Carbohydrates: 4g; Fiber: 0g; Net Carbs: 4g; Protein: 17g; Sugar Alcohols: 0g
Macros: Fat 76% Carbs 4% Protein 19%

Mary's Cinnamon Rolls

VEGETARIAN

Prep time: 30 minutes, plus 30 minutes to chill | **Cook time:** 15 minutes | **Rolls:** 12

I consider cinnamon rolls the holy grail of breakfast comfort food. Just the thought of them makes my mouth water! The aroma of their sticky, gooey greatness coming from the oven always make mornings feel so special, warm, and cozy. These are now a staple in our freezer. I'll make a big batch in advance and then pop a few in the oven as a quick breakfast or to serve on any occasion.

FOR THE DOUGH

Butter or nonstick cooking spray, for greasing
½ cup coconut flour
2 tablespoons granulated erythritol blend
1 teaspoon baking powder
1 teaspoon cinnamon
Pinch salt
2 cups grated mozzarella cheese
5 tablespoons cream cheese
1 large egg

FOR THE FILLING

5 tablespoons cold butter, cubed
¼ cup brown erythritol blend
1 tablespoon cinnamon
1½ teaspoons coconut flour

FOR THE ICING

4 tablespoons cream cheese
2 tablespoons butter
2 tablespoons sugar-free almond milk or milk of your choice
½ cup confectioners' erythritol blend
½ teaspoon vanilla extract

1. Preheat the oven to 400°F, and lightly grease a pie pan with butter or non-stick cooking spray.

2. **To make the dough:** In a small bowl, combine the flour, sweetener, baking powder, cinnamon, and salt. Mix with a fork, mashing out all lumps.

CONTINUED

3. In a large microwave-safe bowl, slowly melt the mozzarella and cream cheese, 30 seconds at a time, until the mozzarella is completely melted. Remove from the microwave and stir until smooth. Add the flour mixture, stir, and then stir in the egg. Using your hands, work the dough to form a ball.

4. Lay the ball on a piece of parchment paper. Using your hands, mash it down to begin making a rectangle. Lay another piece of parchment paper on top, and use a rolling pin or side of a drinking glass to roll the dough ¼ inch thick. Take the top parchment paper off, and with your fingers, work the edges to make them straight. Put a clean parchment paper on top and flip the dough over. Peel the top piece of parchment paper off.

5. **To make the filling:** In a small bowl, use your fingers to mix together the cubed butter, brown sweetener, cinnamon, and flour into a paste. Using a knife, spread it evenly over the dough.

6. With a long end of the dough in front of you, use your fingers and palm of your hand to begin rolling the dough away from you into a tight log. Use the parchment paper to help you roll. Wrap the dough in a fresh piece of parchment paper, and place in the freezer for 30 minutes to an hour.

7. Remove the log from the freezer, and using a serrated knife, cut the log into 12 slices. Arrange the slices side by side in the greased pie pan, and cook for 12 to 15 minutes, or until golden brown.

8. **To make the icing:** Using an electric mixer, mix the cream cheese, butter, milk, confectioners' blend, and vanilla until creamy.

9. Allow the cinnamon rolls to cool for about 5 minutes, and then spread or pipe the icing over the rolls. Cut and serve.

PREP TIP
Keep your hands damp when working with the dough so it won't stick to your fingers as much. If your dough sticks to the parchment paper at any time, put another piece on top and flip it over onto a new piece. A new piece of parchment paper really helps.

Per Serving (1 roll): Calories: 189; Total Fat: 16g; Carbohydrates: 15.5g; Fiber: 2.5g; Net Carbs: 2g; Protein: 6g; Sugar Alcohols: 11g
Macros: Fat 76% Carbs 4% Protein 13%

Raspberry Lemonade

DAIRY-FREE, NUT-FREE, VEGAN

Prep time: 15 minutes | **Cook time:** 45 minutes | **Servings:** 8 (8-ounce)

I've always loved pink lemonade. It looks so fresh and pretty, especially with the lemon wedge on the side. I'm also a lover of raspberries, so I put these two together to make the perfect fancy Mother's Day drink. It's delightful served over ice, but you could also spike it with some vodka and add a sweetener rim if you wanted to take it up a notch or two!

2 cups raspberries, divided

5 to 6 cups water, divided

1 cup freshly squeezed lemon juice (4 to 6 lemons), plus lemon wedges for garnish

1 cup confectioners' erythritol blend

1. Place 1 cup of raspberries in a blender with 1 cup of water, and puree until smooth. To remove all the seeds, pour the mixture into a strainer, and using the back of a spoon, push through the strainer and into a 2-quart pitcher.

2. Add 4 cups of water, lemon juice, and confectioners' blend, and stir well. Add additional water or sweetener to taste.

3. Serve the lemonade in tall glasses over ice with 5 or 6 extra raspberries added in with the ice and on top. Add a wedge of lemon on the side and a paper straw.

SWAP IT
Substitute any other berries for this drink or use a combination of berries. They're all great.

Per Serving: Calories: 23; Total Fat: 0g; Carbohydrates: 21g; Fiber: 2g; Net Carbs: 4g; Protein: 0g; Sugar Alcohols: 15g
Macros: Fat 0% Carbs 70% Protein 0%

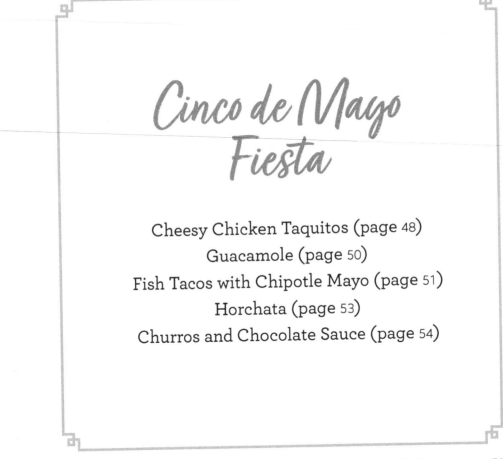

Cinco de Mayo Fiesta

Cheesy Chicken Taquitos (page 48)
Guacamole (page 50)
Fish Tacos with Chipotle Mayo (page 51)
Horchata (page 53)
Churros and Chocolate Sauce (page 54)

Fish Tacos with Chipotle Mayo, page 51

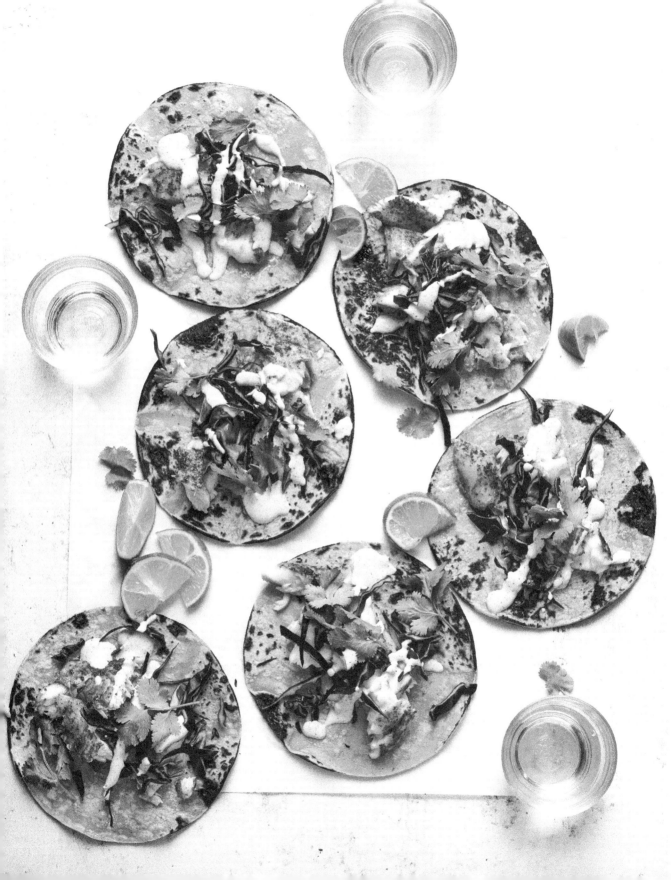

Cheesy Chicken Taquitos

NUT-FREE

Prep time: 15 minutes | **Cook time:** 45 minutes | **Taquitos:** 12

Years ago, my friends and I would hang out at Vernon's in Addison, Texas, and watch all the sporting events. They had taquitos on their appetizer menu, and we'd order two or three batches between us. On many occasions, I would even take an order home. When I started keto, it was one of those foods I figured was off the menu for good, but this keto-fied version is a staple comfort food at our house. Swap the cheddar for another cheese, or switch the chicken for any meat you like. Try them dipped in Guacamole (page 50)!

12 large (deli-sliced) slices cheddar cheese

3 ounces (6 tablespoons) cream cheese

¼ cup tomato salsa

1 tablespoon fresh lime juice

1 teaspoon chili powder

1 teaspoon garlic salt

½ teaspoon freshly ground black pepper

2 cups cooked shredded chicken

¾ cup sour cream

1 or 2 scallions, chopped, for garnish

1. Preheat the oven to 375°F, and line two baking sheets with parchment paper. Lay 6 pieces of cheddar cheese on each baking sheet an equal distance apart.

2. In a medium skillet over medium heat, mix together the cream cheese, salsa, lime juice, chili powder, garlic salt, and pepper. Add the shredded chicken, and mix until heated through. Set aside.

3. Place the baking sheets in the oven for 6 to 10 minutes, or until the edges are brown and the cheese is bubbly. Remove the sheets from the oven and allow to cool for a couple of minutes (see tip). When cool enough to handle, peel the cheese off the parchment paper and place on a clean piece of parchment paper.

4. Spoon 1/12 of the chicken mixture onto each piece of cheese and wrap tightly. Place the taquitos on a serving dish, top each with 1 tablespoon of sour cream, and sprinkle with scallions to garnish.

COOKING TIP

When the cheese comes out of the oven, it needs to be cool enough to handle, but you also need to work quickly because it will harden as it cools. If you double this recipe, you'll want to do it in two batches.

Per Serving (1 taquito): Calories: 177; Total Fat: 13g; Carbohydrates: 2g; Fiber: 0g; Net Carbs: 2g; Protein: 12g; Sugar Alcohols: 0g
Macros: Fat 66% Carbs 5% Protein 27%

Guacamole

DAIRY-FREE, NUT-FREE, VEGAN

Prep time: 15 minutes | **Servings:** 9

I'm somewhat of a self-proclaimed avocado connoisseur. I enjoyed guacamole long before I found keto, and now that I follow this lifestyle, guacamole is front and center for all occasions and included in a majority of my meals. There's not much difference between my pre-keto recipe and the way I make it now—simple and delicious. I prepare mine with a bowl and a fork, but if you have a *molcajete* (mortar and pestle), that's even better. Enjoy this guac with the Cheesy Chicken Taquitos on page 48, the "scoops" (page 136), or top a burger with it!

5 ripe avocados

1 Roma tomato, diced

½ small red onion, finely diced

2 garlic cloves, diced

1 tablespoon lime juice

1 teaspoon salt

½ teaspoon freshly ground black pepper

1 tablespoon minced fresh cilantro, for garnish

Cut the avocados in half, discard the pits and peel off the skin, and put them in a large bowl. Using a fork, mash the avocados. Add the tomato, onion, garlic, lime juice, salt, and pepper. Mix well, and serve garnished with cilantro.

PREP TIP

In the rare event that you have leftover guacamole, put it in a resealable container, and use a spoon to mash it down evenly on top. Add a thin layer of water to the top of the guacamole, put the lid on it, and store it in the refrigerator. Water is the perfect barrier against oxygen and will keep your guacamole perfect and fresh.

Per Serving (⅓ cup): Calories: 131; Total Fat: 12g; Carbohydrates: 8g; Fiber: 5.5g; Net Carbs: 2.5g; Protein: 2g; Sugar Alcohols: 0g
Macros: Fat 82% Carbs 8% Protein 6%

Fish Tacos with Chipotle Mayo

Prep time: 15 minutes | **Cook time:** 30 minutes | **Servings:** 6

I love fish tacos! They always make a beautiful presentation and deliver sensational taste and crunch. You can use any seasonings you'd like, but for Cinco de Mayo, it's got to be spicy so we're using my favorite for both the fish and the mayo—chipotle chili powder! I like tilapia for this dish, but you could also use salmon, cod, or snapper. You can use any cheese you like for the taco shells. Or, if they work for your macros, you can use low carb tortillas instead.

1 cup mayonnaise

2 tablespoons water

2 teaspoons lime juice

½ teaspoon chipotle chili powder

2 pounds tilapia

2 tablespoons olive oil

1 tablespoon chipotle chili powder

12 large mozzarella cheese slices

2 cups shredded red cabbage

Cilantro, for garnish

2 limes, cut into wedges, for squeezing

1. Preheat the oven to 425°F, and line a baking sheet with parchment paper.

2. In a small bowl, make the chipotle mayo by mixing together the mayonnaise, water, lime juice, and chipotle chili powder. Place in a serving bowl or squirt bottle, and set aside.

3. Rub the tilapia fillets with the olive oil, dust with the chipotle chili powder, and bake on the lined baking sheet for 10 to 12 minutes, or until flaky. Remove from the oven and set aside. Once cool, roughly chop the fish and place in a serving bowl.

4. Reduce the oven temperature to 350°F, and line a baking sheet with parchment paper. Place 6 mozzarella cheese slices on the baking sheet. Bake for 5 to 7 minutes, until the edges are brown and the cheese is bubbly.

CONTINUED

5. While the cheese is cooking, set up three kitchen spatulas or wooden spoons, each one suspended between two glasses.

6. Remove the tray from the oven and wait a couple of minutes until the cheese is cool enough to handle. Using a spatula without slots, pick up three slices of cheese and drape them over the spoons. They will quickly cool into hard taco shells. Once cooled, place to the side, and repeat with the remaining three cheese slices.

7. Bake the remaining 6 cheese slices for 5 to 7 minutes, and form into taco shells like in step 6.

8. Load the taco shells with fish, shredded cabbage, and a drizzle of chipotle mayonnaise, and garnish with cilantro. Serve with lime wedges for squeezing.

PREP TIP

Don't worry if you forgot to thaw the fish. Simply prepare the fish frozen, and add 10 to 15 minutes to your cooking time.

Per Serving (2 tacos): Calories: 613; Total Fat: 46g; Carbohydrates: 5g; Fiber: 1g; Net Carbs: 4g; Protein: 45g; Sugar Alcohols: 0g
Macros: Fat 68% Carbs 3% Protein 29%

Horchata

DAIRY-FREE, VEGAN

Prep time: 5 minutes | **Servings:** 4 (8-ounce)

Ever had a horchata? Oh my goodness, it is amazing. It's like drinking a glass of milk leftover from cinnamon toast cereal. As soon as I took the first sip of the real thing, I knew immediately how to make it keto. It's such a festive drink, perfect for celebrating Cinco de Mayo or any occasion. Simply poured over ice it's wonderful, but you could really set it free with a shot of vodka or add some ice to the blender and serve it frozen.

4 cups sugar-free vanilla almond milk or sugar-free coconut milk

½ cup granulated erythritol blend

2 tablespoons brown erythritol blend

1½ teaspoons cinnamon, plus extra for garnish

1 teaspoon vanilla

In a blender, combine the milk, sweetener, brown sweetener, cinnamon, and vanilla. Blend for one minute. Pour over ice, sprinkle a little cinnamon on top, and serve.

SPICE IT UP

To make this drink a little fancier, place a cinnamon stick in the glass, and cut a strawberry halfway up the middle and hang it on the edge.

Per Serving: Calories: 32; Total Fat: 2.5g; Carbohydrates: 32g; Fiber: 1.5g; Net Carbs: 0.5g; Protein: 1g; Sugar Alcohols: 30g
Macros: Fat 70% Carbs 6% Protein 13%

Churros and Chocolate Sauce

VEGETARIAN

Prep time: 20 minutes | **Cook time:** 10 minutes | **Servings:** 9

These delicious morsels have been available at every fair and event I've attended for as long as I can remember. If you didn't see the booth right away, the smell wafting through the park and the sight of others carrying their churro-filled paper boats meant these cinnamon sugar fritters were somewhere close. After several attempts, I got the keto version just right and came up with what I think is greatness. They're crispy on the outside, soft on the inside—perfect on their own, but, hey, it's Cinco de Mayo, so I added some chocolate sauce for dipping! Because we're using such a large amount of oil for deep-frying, I'm using peanut oil instead of coconut or avocado oil because it's much less expensive.

FOR THE CHURROS

8 cups peanut oil, for frying

½ cup almond flour

½ cup whey protein isolate, unflavored

¼ cup coconut flour

½ teaspoon psyllium husk powder

2 tablespoons granulated erythritol blend

3 large eggs

2 tablespoons olive oil

1 teaspoon vanilla extract

1 cup monk fruit granulated erythritol blend

1 teaspoon cinnamon

FOR THE CHOCOLATE SAUCE

½ cup heavy cream

½ cup unsweetened almond milk

½ cup confectioners' erythritol blend

½ cup unsweetened cocoa powder

1 teaspoon vanilla extract

½ teaspoon cinnamon

1. Place a large, heavy pot on the stove over medium heat. Pour enough peanut oil in the pot to fill at least ¾ inch to 1 inch deep.

2. **To make the churros:** In a large bowl, combine the almond flour, whey protein, coconut flour, psyllium husk powder, and sweetener. Stir well with a spoon, mashing up any lumps. Add the eggs, olive oil, and vanilla, and mix well.

3. Spoon the dough into a piping bag or gallon resealable bag with the corner cut off to make a ½-inch hole.

4. In a shallow bowl, mix the sweetener and cinnamon to make the rolling sugar.

5. When the oil is hot enough to fry (see tip on page 21), pipe 3 lines of dough into the oil 4 to 5 inches long. Using a slotted spoon, flip the churros back and forth in the oil for 2 to 4 minutes, or until golden brown. Carefully lift each one out of the oil and place in the rolling sugar. Spoon the sugar across the top of each churro, and then move them to a plate. Repeat cooking and coating with the remaining batter.

6. **To make the chocolate sauce:** Heat a small pot over medium heat. Combine the heavy cream, almond milk, confectioners' sweetener, cocoa powder, vanilla, and cinnamon in the pan, and whisk or stir until it comes to a boil. Reduce heat to a simmer and continue to stir for 5 more minutes. Remove from heat, and continue stirring a few minutes more while the sauce thickens. Pour the sauce in a dish for dipping, and serve with the churros.

SPICE IT UP

I use a piping bag with the Ateco tip #824, but you could also use the Wilton 1M tip. Learn more about these on page 19. You'll use them many times in your baking and decorating adventures.

Per Serving (2 churros and 2 tablespoons chocolate sauce): Calories: 308; Total Fat: 25g; Carbohydrates: 38g; Fiber: 4g; Net Carbs: 3g; Protein: 16g; Sugar Alcohols: 31g
Macros: Fat 73% Carbs 4% Protein 21%

CHAPTER FOUR

Summer Celebrations

Summer seems like it was created for celebrating, don't you think? Warm, sunny weather, long days, starry nights, and a whole lot of outdoor cooking! I'm serving up the recipes that exemplify the free-spiritedness of the season—from a Father's Day feast for the special dad in your life to a luscious summertime cookout and a Fourth of July picnic studded with patriotic favorites. Tuck in that napkin and let's get started!

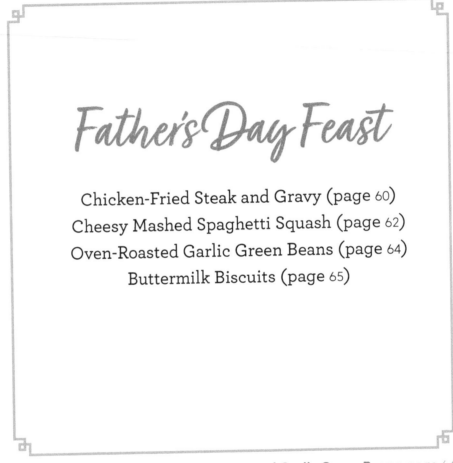

Father's Day Feast

Chicken-Fried Steak and Gravy (page 60)

Cheesy Mashed Spaghetti Squash (page 62)

Oven-Roasted Garlic Green Beans (page 64)

Buttermilk Biscuits (page 65)

Oven-Roasted Garlic Green Beans, page 64

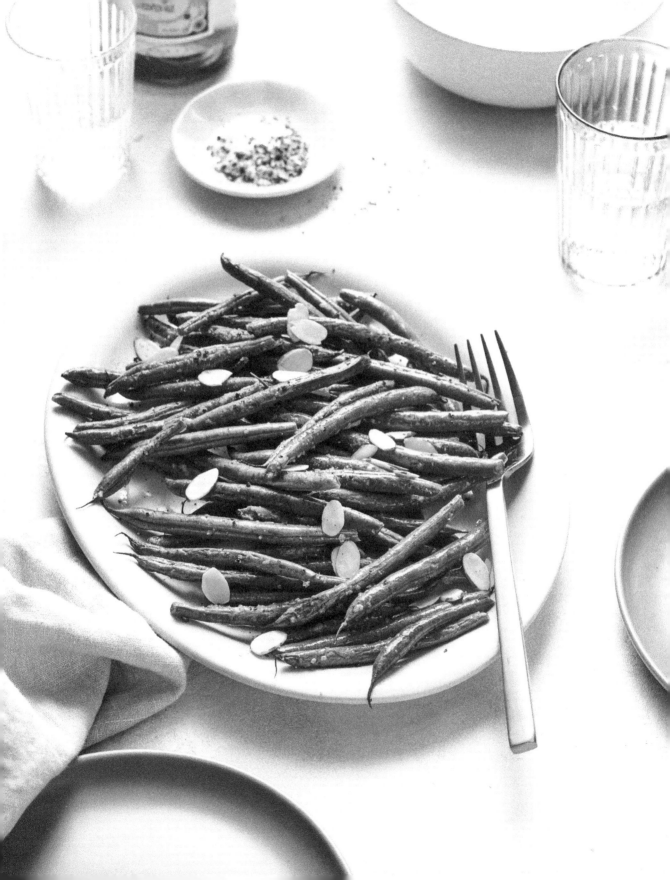

Chicken-Fried Steak and Gravy

Prep time: 30 minutes | Cook time: 30 minutes | Servings: 6

National Chicken Fried Steak Day is in October, but here in Texas, chicken-fried steak is an essential food and deeply embedded tradition that we celebrate every day we can. Covered in cream gravy, this steak may be the most popular comfort food ever, especially with the men in my life! You start off with a cheap piece of meat, pound it out, hand-batter it, deep-fry it, and then cover it in cream gravy. It used to be my guilty pleasure, but now that I've made it keto-friendly, we're able to enjoy it all the time without guilt. Save your next batch of bacon or sausage grease from breakfast, and you can make the gravy anytime!

FOR THE CHICKEN-FRIED STEAK

3 cups lard or coconut or avocado oil, for frying

6 (4-ounce) cube steaks (1½ pounds total)

2 teaspoons salt, divided

1⅓ cups whey protein isolate, unflavored

1 teaspoon freshly ground black pepper

1 teaspoon garlic powder

1 teaspoon baking powder

1 teaspoon baking soda

½ cup buttermilk

½ cup almond milk

2 large eggs

FOR THE CREAM GRAVY

¼ cup lard or oil reserved from frying

1 cup heavy cream

½ cup almond milk

¾ teaspoon xanthan gum

⅛ teaspoon salt

⅛ teaspoon freshly ground black pepper

1. Place a large, heavy skillet on the stove, and fill with the lard or oil.

2. **To make the chicken-fried steak:** Place a cube steak between two pieces of plastic wrap. Using a mallet, pound the steak out to less than ¼ inch thick. Remove the plastic wrap, sprinkle with ¼ teaspoon of salt, set aside, and repeat with the remaining steaks.

3. Place two shallow bowls on the counter next to the stove. In one bowl, combine the whey protein, remaining ½ teaspoon of salt, pepper, and garlic powder, and mix well. In the other bowl, combine the baking powder and baking soda, mix them together, and then whisk in the buttermilk, almond milk, and eggs.

4. Over medium heat, heat the oil to 350°F (see page 21 for tip if you don't have a thermometer). Place one of the steaks in the whey protein mixture and press down all over to coat, flip over, and repeat. Place the steak in the egg mixture, turn to coat both sides, and then transfer back over to the whey protein mixture. Using the back of a spoon, mash the steak down on each side to fully coat.

5. Carefully lay the steak in the hot lard or oil. When the edges are golden brown, use tongs to flip, and cook for another 3 minutes. Remove from the pan, place on paper towels, and cover loosely with aluminum foil to keep warm. Repeat coating and frying, one steak at a time. Once all the steaks are fried, turn off the heat and allow the lard or oil to cool for 5 to 10 minutes. Discard the oil, reserving ¼ cup to go back in the pan.

6. **To make the cream gravy:** Reduce heat to medium-low, and add the lard or oil. Heat for 2 minutes, and then add the heavy cream and almond milk. Stir continuously. When the milk begins to bubble, add the xanthan gum, salt, and pepper, and stir vigorously or whisk. When it begins to thicken, reduce heat and keep stirring. If it gets too thick, stir in a little more almond milk. Serve steaks topped with warm gravy.

PREP TIP

This dish isn't like traditional chicken-fried steak where you can batter and lay them aside. This batter comes off easily, so make sure you're only battering and frying one steak at a time. Also, really watch the lard or oil so it doesn't get too hot and burn your steaks. If you see it beginning to smoke, turn down the heat.

Per Serving (1 steak and ¼ cup gravy): Calories: 575; Total Fat: 37g; Carbohydrates: 3.5g; Fiber: 0.5g; Net Carbs: 3g; Protein: 55g; Sugar Alcohols: 0g
Macros: Fat 58% Carbs 2% Protein 38%

Cheesy Mashed Spaghetti Squash

NUT-FREE

Prep time: 20 minutes | **Cook time:** 1 hour | **Servings:** 8

Spaghetti squash is easy to cook and so versatile in recipes. This recipe is one of the easiest of all and absolutely delicious. It's also one of Lovies's favorites, so we fix it a lot at my house. Wonderfully cheesy with a mashed potato vibe, this comfort food is great by itself as a side or as a full-blown meal with some chopped grilled or rotisserie chicken.

Oil or nonstick cooking spray, for greasing

1 small spaghetti squash, about 2 pounds

1 tablespoon olive oil

1½ teaspoon salt, divided

8 ounces (1 brick) cream cheese

½ cup heavy cream

½ cup chicken broth

½ teaspoon freshly ground black pepper

½ teaspoon garlic powder

½ cup grated Gruyère or Swiss cheese

½ cup grated Parmesan cheese, divided

Chives, for garnish

1. Preheat the oven to 425°F, and line a baking sheet with parchment paper. Lightly grease a 2-quart baking dish or pan and set aside.

2. Cut the spaghetti squash in half lengthwise. With a spoon, scoop out all the seeds and fibers. Drizzle the inside of each half with the olive oil, season with ½ teaspoon of salt, and lay flat-side down on the lined baking sheet. Bake for 30 minutes, turn the squash over, and bake for 5 more minutes. Remove from the oven, and allow to cool for 5 to 10 minutes.

3. Using a fork, rake the squash strands into a small colander or cheesecloth. Mash or squeeze out as much of the excess water as you can, and then place the squash in the baking dish.

4. In a blender, combine the cream cheese, heavy cream, broth, remaining ½ teaspoon of salt, pepper, and garlic powder. Pulse 2 or 3 times until smooth, and pour into the baking dish on top of the spaghetti squash. Add the Gruyère cheese and ¼ cup of Parmesan cheese, and stir until completely mixed.

5. Reduce the oven temperature to 350°F. Bake the casserole for 40 minutes. Remove from the oven, sprinkle with the remaining ¼ cup of Parmesan, and cook another 5 minutes, until golden brown. Remove from the oven, and garnish with chives.

SPICE IT UP

For a little extra flavor and to add some color, add some thin slices of roasted red onions and bacon to the cream cheese mixture.

Per Serving: Calories: 250; Total Fat: 22g; Carbohydrates: 8g; Fiber: 1g; Net Carbs: 7g; Protein: 6g; Sugar Alcohols: 0g
Macros: Fat 79% Carbs 11% Protein 10%

Oven-Roasted Garlic Green Beans

DAIRY-FREE, NUT-FREE, VEGAN

Prep time: 15 minutes | **Cook time:** 15 minutes | **Servings:** 6

Green beans have graced our family's table on every occasion as far back as I can remember. They're the kind of dish that everyone loves, and they pair well with whatever you're serving. This roasted version may be my favorite, although I've never met a green bean dish I didn't love.

1½ pounds green beans, ends trimmed

3 tablespoons olive oil

6 cloves garlic, minced

1 teaspoon salt

½ teaspoon freshly ground black pepper

1. Preheat the oven to 400°F, and line a baking sheet with parchment paper.
2. Combine the beans and olive oil in a gallon resealable bag. Seal the bag, gently flip and shake until all the beans are coated, and then empty and scatter the beans on the parchment paper. Top with the minced garlic, and season with the salt and pepper.
3. Roast for 12 to 15 minutes, or until slightly brown and tender, shaking the tray halfway through. Watch them, as they will brown up fast.

SPICE IT UP
To dress the dish up a bit, sprinkle some fresh grated Parmesan or slivered almonds across the top after roasting.

Per Serving: Calories: 95; Total Fat: 7g; Carbohydrates: 8g; Fiber: 3g; Net Carbs: 5g; Protein: 2g; Sugar Alcohols: 0g
Macros: Fat 66% Carbs 21% Protein 8%

Buttermilk Biscuits

VEGETARIAN

Prep time: 15 minutes | **Cook time:** 15 minutes | **Biscuits:** 8

Bread has always been my weakness, especially buttermilk biscuits. I can vividly remember as a child getting so excited to crack open the can and place them carefully on the cookie sheet. The smell was intoxicating and would make your nose lift and your eyes close as you took it all in. When I started keto, biscuits were one of the first things I tried to keto-fy. I've made many versions over the years, but this is the keeper.

Oil or nonstick cooking spray, for greasing

½ cup almond flour

½ cup coconut flour

2 teaspoons granulated erythritol blend

1 teaspoon baking powder

½ teaspoon baking soda

¼ teaspoon salt

5 large eggs

½ teaspoons cream of tartar

¼ cup buttermilk

2 tablespoons cold butter, cubed, plus melted butter for brushing

1 tablespoon olive oil

1. Preheat the oven to 400°F, and grease a standard muffin pan.

2. In a medium bowl, combine the almond flour, coconut flour, sweetener, baking powder, baking soda, and salt. Mix well to mash out any lumps.

3. Separate the eggs, and put the yolks in the flour mixture and the whites in another bowl. To the bowl with the egg whites, add the cream of tartar, and with an electric mixer, whip on high until stiff peaks form, about a minute.

4. To the flour mixture, add the buttermilk, cold butter, and olive oil, and use your hands to mix and mash until fully incorporated.

5. Add the egg whites to the flour mixture, and gently cut and fold over and over, until the whites are worked into the dough. It will be a little lumpy.

6. Drop spoonfuls of dough evenly into 8 muffin holes, and bake for 10 minutes. Remove from the oven, brush with melted butter, and cook 5 additional minutes, or until golden brown.

Per Serving (1 biscuit): Calories: 164; Total Fat: 13g; Carbohydrates: 6.5g; Fiber: 3.5g; Net Carbs: 2g; Protein: 7g; Sugar Alcohols: 1g
Macros: Fat 71% Carbs 5% Protein 17%

Summer Cookout

Smoked Ribs (page 68)

Bacon Barbecued Chicken (page 69)

Bacon and Egg Cheeseburgers (page 70)

Grilled Avocados (page 72)

Jalapeño Ranch Creamy Coleslaw (page 73)

Apple Pie Bites (page 74)

Smoked Ribs, page 68

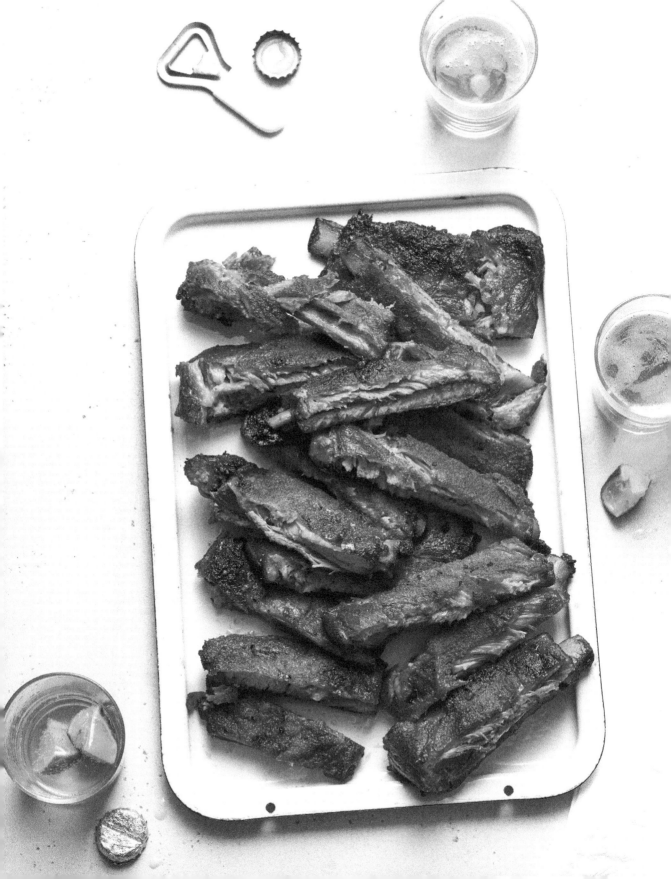

Smoked Ribs

NUT-FREE

Prep time: 20 minutes, plus 5 hours to chill | **Cook time:** 5 hours | **Servings:** 8

It wouldn't be barbecue season without ribs, and my favorite is St. Louis–style pork ribs. They're large and meaty with a big bone, meaning lots of fat for added flavor. I can eat an entire rack on my own and often do. Here in Texas, the tradition is to cook them low and slow without sauce, but you do what makes you happy. Have some paper towels close by—these ribs get messy!

¼ cup brown erythritol blend

1 tablespoon paprika

1 tablespoon Lawry's seasoned salt

1 tablespoon garlic powder

1 tablespoon freshly ground black pepper

4 racks (8 to 10 pounds) St. Louis–style pork ribs, trimmed

¼ cup (½ stick) butter, melted

1. In a small bowl, combine the brown sweetener, paprika, seasoned salt, garlic powder, and pepper. Set aside.

2. Remove the ribs from the packaging, and using a knife, carefully remove the thin membrane on the bony side. Using a spoon, sprinkle the rub on the ribs, and then, using the back of the spoon as a mallet, slowly and gently pound the rub all over each rack so it sticks. Wrap each rack in plastic wrap and refrigerate for at least 5 to 6 hours or up to overnight.

3. Preheat a grill or smoker to 180°F. Unwrap and lay each rack directly on the racks, meaty-side up, and cook for 2 hours.

4. Remove the ribs, and increase heat to 250°F. Place each rack on a large sheet of aluminum foil. Pour the melted butter over each rack, wrap tightly in the foil, and place back in the heat for 3 more hours. Serve warm.

COOKING TIP

To make these in the oven, line a baking sheet with aluminum foil or parchment paper. Place a baking rack on the baking sheet, and then put the ribs on the rack, meaty-side up. Broil for 5 minutes, and then reduce the oven to 300°F and cook for 1½ hours. Cover with foil and cook another 1½ hours until a knife slides into the meat easily.

Per Serving (½ rack): Calories: 903; Total Fat: 79g; Carbohydrates: 6g; Fiber: 0g; Net Carbs: 0g; Protein: 49g; Sugar Alcohols: 6g
Macros: Fat 79% Carbs 0% Protein 22%

Bacon Barbecued Chicken

DAIRY-FREE, NUT-FREE

Prep time: 15 minutes | **Cook time:** 15 minutes | **Servings:** 8

This chicken is pounded thin, slathered in barbecue sauce, rolled up with bacon, and then grilled, making every single bite amazing. It's perfect for a warm summer night with friends and family out by the pool, and if you have any left over, it's equally tasty the next day chopped up in a salad.

8 (6-ounce) skinless boneless chicken breasts

½ cup brown erythritol blend

½ cup soy sauce

3 tablespoons olive oil

1 teaspoon garlic powder

½ teaspoon freshly ground black pepper

16 slices bacon

1. Preheat the grill to medium-high heat. Soak 16 toothpicks in water.

2. Place a chicken breast between two large pieces of plastic wrap and use a rolling pin or mallet to pound to ¼-inch thickness. Repeat with the remaining chicken breasts.

3. In a small bowl, mix together the brown sweetener, soy sauce, olive oil, garlic powder, and pepper. Rub or brush half of the mixture onto both sides of the breasts.

4. Roll up a chicken breast and wrap with two slices of bacon, end to end, secured with toothpicks. Brush more of the soy sauce mixture on the bacon, and repeat with the remaining breasts.

5. Place the chicken on the grill, seam-side down, and grill for 6 to 8 minutes on each side, or until cooked through. Remove from grill, let sit for a few minutes, and then serve.

COOKING TIP

You can also bake these in the oven at 350°F for about 40 minutes. Check to see if the chicken is done by cutting into it—if it's pink, it needs a little more time.

Per Serving: Calories: 487; Total Fat: 28g; Carbohydrates: 14g; Fiber: 0g; Net Carbs: 2g; Protein: 54g; Sugar Alcohols: 12g
Macros: Fat 52% Carbs 2% Protein 44%

Bacon and Egg Cheeseburgers

NUT-FREE

Prep time: 15 minutes, plus 2 hours to chill | **Cook time:** 25 minutes | **Servings:** 8

When summer rolls around, there's nothing better than cooking burgers on the grill. They always taste great with a slice of cheese, but the real pièce de résistance is the egg we'll top them with. The runny yolk mixed with the cheese and meat is like a little slice of heaven—so good! If you like, you can also add avocado slices, tomato, and onion or serve the burgers over a bed of lettuce and turn the dish into a salad.

4 pounds ground beef

1 teaspoon salt

1 teaspoon freshly ground black pepper

2 tablespoons olive oil, for brushing the burgers

8 large (deli-sliced) slices cheddar cheese

Butter or nonstick cooking spray, for greasing

8 large eggs

8 slices bacon, cooked until crispy

Paprika, for garnish

1. In a large bowl, mix together the ground beef, salt, and pepper. Divide the ground beef into 8 sections, roll each into a ball and pat into a ¾-inch-thick patty. Press your thumb in the middle of each patty to make a divot, and place on a tray. Cover with plastic wrap or foil, and refrigerate for at least 2 hours or up to overnight.

2. When ready to cook, heat the grill to high. Brush the burgers with the olive oil on both sides.

3. Cook on the first side for 3 minutes, and then flip and cook 4 more minutes. Add the slices of cheese, and then cook another minute. For medium-rare, cook 1 minute less, and for well done, cook 1 minute more.

4. While the burgers are cooking, generously grease a standard muffin pan with butter or nonstick spray, and crack an egg into 8 of the muffin holes. Place the muffin pan on the grill after you flip the burger and cook for 2 minutes; then remove from heat.

5. Plate the cheeseburgers, and top each one with a slice of crispy bacon. Use a spoon to scoop the eggs out of the muffin pan, and place one on top of each burger. Garnish with paprika, and serve.

COOKING TIP

The burgers can also be cooked in a cast-iron pan or in the broiler. But don't flip them back and forth; just the one time is enough. Also, don't press down on the meat while you're cooking. That squeezes out all the good juices you're trying to keep in.

Per Serving: Calories: 616; Total Fat: 42g; Carbohydrates: 0g; Fiber: 0g; Net Carbs: 0g; Protein: 55g; Sugar Alcohols: 0g
Macros: Fat 61% Carbs 0% Protein 36%

Grilled Avocados

DAIRY-FREE, NUT-FREE, VEGAN

Prep time: 5 minutes | **Cook time:** 5 minutes | **Servings:** 8

I'm obsessed with avocados and eat them on just about everything. If you're firing up the grill for a cookout, you've got to try grilled avocados. They taste amazing with the smoky grill flavor, and the presentation is outstanding. I prefer them simple with a little olive oil and salt, but you could get creative and top them with Parmesan cheese or salsa and sour cream, or mash them into smoky guacamole. The possibilities are endless!

4 avocados, cut in half longwise, pitted

4 tablespoons olive oil
1 teaspoon salt

1. Preheat the grill to medium-high heat.
2. Brush or drizzle the olive oil on the cut side of each avocado, and season with the salt.
3. Lay cut-side down, grill 5 minutes, and serve.

COOKING TIP
They won't be as smoky as grilled, but these could also be made in a cast-iron pan on the stovetop.

Per Serving (½ avocado): Calories: 173; Total Fat: 17g; Carbohydrates: 5.5g; Fiber: 4.5g; Net Carbs: 1g; Protein: 1g; Sugar Alcohols: 0g
Macros: Fat 88% Carbs 2% Protein 2%

Jalapeño Ranch Creamy Coleslaw

NUT-FREE, VEGETARIAN

Prep time: 10 minutes, plus 1 hour to chill | **Servings:** 8

This coleslaw recipe is a crowd-pleaser and one of our favorites. The dressing reminds me of the jalapeño ranch served at Chuy's, a popular restaurant near me, and that alone is fantastic, but when it's added to cabbage, all the crunch makes it the perfect side dish. It's easy to make the dressing in advance, and then all you do is open a package of cabbage, add the dressing, and toss. If it's half the hit for you that it is for me, you'll have two or three extra bags of cabbage waiting and ready to go at any given time.

1 (16-ounce) bag coleslaw mix or cabbage

1 (1-ounce) package ranch dressing mix

1 cup mayonnaise

¾ cup sour cream

2 scallions, thinly sliced

¼ cup jalapeño juice, from a jar

1 jalapeño, seeded and chopped

1. Empty the coleslaw mix into a large serving bowl.

2. In a medium bowl, combine the ranch dressing mix, mayonnaise, sour cream, scallions, jalapeño juice, and jalapeño. Pour 1 cup of the dressing over the coleslaw mix, and toss until mixed.

3. Allow to refrigerate for at least an hour or up to overnight, and serve. Store the extra dressing in the refrigerator (see tip).

PAIR IT

This recipe purposefully makes extra dressing. Use it for dipping raw vegetables, lettuce salads, pizza, and anything else you want to dip or drizzle. It's absolutely delicious on everything.

Per Serving (1½ cups coleslaw with dressing): Calories: 264; Total Fat: 24g; Carbohydrates: 8g; Fiber: 1.5g; Net Carbs: 6.5g; Protein: 2g; Sugar Alcohols: 0g
Macros: Fat 82% Carbs 10% Protein 3%

Per Serving (2 tablespoons dressing only): Calories: 139; Total Fat: 14g; Carbohydrates: 2g; Fiber: 0g; Net Carbs: 2g; Protein: 1g; Sugar Alcohols: 0g
Macros: Fat 91% Carbs 6% Protein 3%

Apple Pie Bites

NUT-FREE, VEGETARIAN

Prep time: 15 minutes | **Cook time:** 25 minutes | **Servings:** 12

When it comes to summer cookouts, you can't beat apple pie. This all-American dessert never disappoints. The outer crust with the gooey apple filling and a hint of cinnamon is absolutely scrumptious and makes the perfect bite-size treat. These bites are a big hit at my cookouts and keep me on the guest list when I show up with a loaded tray to share!

FOR THE CRUST

Oil or nonstick cooking spray, for greasing

¾ cup grated mozzarella cheese

1 ounce (2 tablespoons) cream cheese

3 tablespoons coconut flour

1 tablespoon granulated erythritol blend

FOR THE FILLING

1 small jicama, peeled and chopped into ¼-inch cubes (about 2 cups)

3 tablespoons butter

2 tablespoons water

3 tablespoons brown erythritol blend

1 teaspoon cinnamon

1 teaspoon apple pie spice

½ teaspoon vanilla extract

1. Preheat the oven to 300°F, and grease a mini muffin pan.

2. **To make the crust:** In a small microwave-safe bowl, slowly melt the mozzarella cheese and cream cheese in 20-second increments until the mozzarella is smooth. Remove from the microwave, and stir.

3. Add the flour and sweetener to the cheese mixture, using your hands to work into a dough, and divide into 12 sections. Roll a section into a ball, mash it flat in the palm of your hand, and push into a hole in the muffin pan so that it fills the bottom and sides to make a shell. Repeat with remaining dough.

4. Bake for 8 to 10 minutes, or until golden brown, and then remove from oven and set aside to cool.

5. **To make the filling:** In a small saucepan over medium heat, add the chopped jicama, butter, water, brown sweetener, cinnamon, apple pie spice, and vanilla. Cook for 8 to 10 minutes, stirring often, until the jicama softens.

6. Remove the shells from the pan. Using a small spoon, fill each shell with the jicama filling, and serve.

SPICE IT UP
For a little extra flavor, add chopped pecans to the filling or top with sugar-free whipped cream (page 114).

Per Serving (1 bite): Calories: 83; Total Fat: 7g; Carbohydrates: 8g; Fiber: 2.5g; Net Carbs: 1.5g; Protein: 2g; Sugar Alcohols: 4g
Macros: Fat 76% Carbs 7% Protein 10%

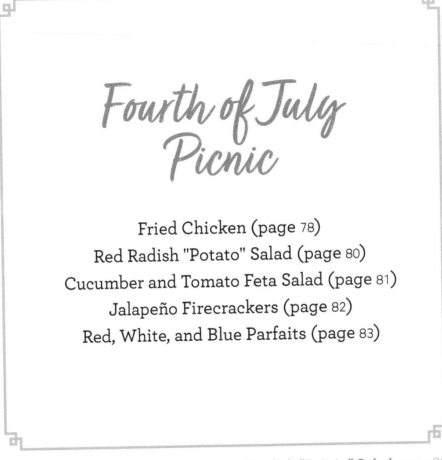

Fourth of July Picnic

Fried Chicken (page 78)
Red Radish "Potato" Salad (page 80)
Cucumber and Tomato Feta Salad (page 81)
Jalapeño Firecrackers (page 82)
Red, White, and Blue Parfaits (page 83)

Red Radish "Potato" Salad, page 80

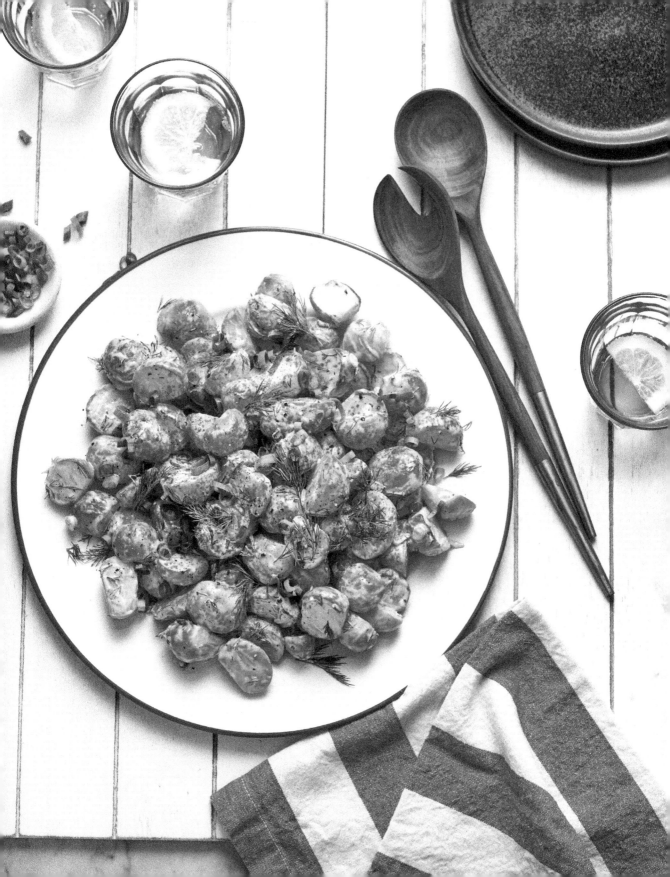

Fried Chicken

Prep time: 15 minutes | **Cook time:** 45 minutes | **Servings:** 8

As a kid, I can remember grabbing some lawn chairs and blankets, piling in the family station wagon, and heading to KFC to grab a big bucket of chicken and all the sides. We'd make our way to the picnic ground, set up camp, and enjoy our feast. This keto-friendly version is crispy on the outside, moist on the inside, and lick-your-fingers good. It reminds me so much of those wonderful days. I make it with bone-in, skin-on thighs, but you can use whatever cut you like. If you have big eaters, you might think about doubling the recipe. Nothing wrong with leftover fried chicken!

3 cups lard, coconut oil, or avocado oil, for frying

8 chicken thighs, bone-in, skin-on (about 3 pounds)

2 teaspoons salt, divided

1½ cups whey protein isolate, unflavored

1 teaspoon garlic powder

1 teaspoon freshly ground black pepper

1 teaspoon baking powder

1 teaspoon baking soda

½ cup buttermilk

½ cup almond milk

3 large eggs

1. Preheat the oven to 325°F, and place a cooling rack on top of a baking sheet.

2. Place a large, heavy skillet on the stove, and fill it with the lard or oil.

3. Season the chicken thighs with 1 teaspoon of salt.

4. Put two shallow bowls on the counter beside the stove. In one bowl, combine the whey protein, garlic powder, remaining teaspoon of salt, and pepper, and mix well. In the other bowl, combine the baking powder and baking soda, and mix together. Add the buttermilk, almond milk, and eggs. Whisk well with a fork.

5. Over medium heat, heat the oil to 350°F. (If you don't have a thermometer, see the tip on page 21.)

6. Place one of the thighs in the whey protein mixture and press down to coat, flip over, and coat, spooning flour on any places not covered. Dredge the thigh in the egg mixture, coating both sides, and then back over to the whey protein mixture. Use the back of a spoon to mash the flour onto the thigh, flip, and mash the other side, spooning flour to fully coat. Pick up the thigh, and carefully lay in the hot oil.

7. When the edges around the thigh are golden brown, use tongs to turn the thigh over and cook 2 or 3 minutes, until golden brown. Transfer the thigh onto the cooling rack on the baking sheet. One at a time, repeat coating and frying with each thigh, and then place the baking sheet in oven to finish cooking for 15 to 20 minutes. Remove from the oven and serve.

COOKING TIP

I always recommend cutting into the chicken to make sure it's cooked clear through. Remove the tray from the oven, pick the largest thigh, and cut into the meatiest part. If there's no pink, it's cooked. If you see pink, cook for a few more minutes.

Per Serving (1 thigh): Calories: 418; Total Fat: 24g; Carbohydrates: 2g; Fiber: 0g; Net Carbs: 2g; Protein: 49g; Sugar Alcohols: 0g
Macros: Fat 52% Carbs 2% Protein 47%

Red Radish "Potato" Salad

NUT-FREE, VEGETARIAN

Prep time: 15 minutes | **Cook time:** 45 minutes | **Servings:** 8

One of my favorite picnic foods is potato salad, which is not keto-friendly. I had pretty much written this dish off until I read a magazine article about roasting radishes and how much they tasted like potatoes. Crisis averted, and "potato" salad is back on the menu! There are many things you can add to this recipe to make it your own, such as chopped pickles or relish, boiled eggs, red onion, celery, and so much more.

4 pounds red radishes, leaves and ends trimmed, halved (about 8 bunches)

4 tablespoons olive oil

1 teaspoon salt

1 teaspoon freshly ground black pepper

1 teaspoon garlic powder

¼ cup heavy cream

1 cup mayonnaise

3 tablespoons chopped dill

1 tablespoon white vinegar

3 scallions, chopped

2 teaspoons Dijon mustard

Paprika, for garnish

1. Preheat the oven to 350°F, and line a baking sheet with parchment paper.

2. In a gallon resealable bag, add the radishes and olive oil. Seal and shake gently to evenly coat. Empty the radishes onto the lined baking sheet, arrange cut-side up, and season with the salt, pepper, and garlic powder. Roast for 45 minutes, shaking the pan occasionally. Remove from the oven, cool, and then transfer to a large serving bowl.

3. In a small bowl, use a hand mixer to whip the heavy cream, mayonnaise, dill, vinegar, scallions, and Dijon mustard. Pour over the radishes, gently fold into the mixture until incorporated, garnish with paprika, and serve.

COOKING TIP

These radishes will be fork-tender in the oven around 25 minutes, but they taste better if you let them roast for about 45 minutes. If they get too brown, pull them out of the oven sooner.

Per Serving: Calories: 300; Total Fat: 30g; Carbohydrates: 6g; Fiber: 2.5g; Net Carbs: 3.5g; Protein: 2g; Sugar Alcohols: 0g
Macros: Fat 90% Carbs 5% Protein 3%

Cucumber and Tomato Feta Salad

NUT-FREE, VEGETARIAN

Prep time: 15 minutes | **Servings:** 8

This recipe is a winner every time I host a party. It's crisp, colorful, and full of flavor. Not to mention, it's so easy to put together and can be made the night before. The homemade dressing knocks it out of the ballpark for flavor, but you could use your favorite vinaigrette recipe instead. If you make it ahead of time, wait to add the dressing until you're ready to serve. If you happen to have leftovers, add some grilled chicken or shrimp for a tasty and quick lunch the next day.

3 medium cucumbers, peeled, cut into ¼-inch-thick slices and then quartered

2 Roma tomatoes, roughly chopped

12 pitted kalamata olives (or your favorite), halved

8 ounces feta cheese, cut into cubes or crumbled

¼ cup chopped red onion

½ cup olive oil

3 tablespoons red wine vinegar

½ teaspoon Dijon mustard

1 teaspoon garlic salt

1 teaspoon freshly ground black pepper

1. In a large serving bowl, combine the cucumbers, tomatoes, olives, feta, and onion.

2. In a small bowl, whisk together the olive oil, vinegar, Dijon mustard, garlic salt, and pepper.

3. Add the dressing to the salad, toss all the ingredients, and serve.

SPICE IT UP
For a fancier presentation, you can peel 4 slices off the cucumber (one on each side) and leave the remaining skin so it looks like stripes. Top the salad with some chopped cilantro or dill.

Per Serving: Calories: 219; Total Fat: 18g; Carbohydrates: 4g; Fiber: 1g; Net Carbs: 3g; Protein: 6g; Sugar Alcohols: 0g
Macros: Fat 74% Carbs 5% Protein 11%

Jalapeño Firecrackers

NUT-FREE

Prep time: 20 minutes | **Cook time:** 20 minutes | **Servings:** 8

Jalapeño cream cheese poppers are a perfect addition to any picnic. For special occasions, I dress them up with sugar-free apricot preserves and red pepper flakes for an extra spicy-sweet kick. Boy do these go fast at my parties!

8 (3- to 4-inch) jalapeños

6 ounces cream cheese

¼ cup sugar-free apricot preserves

⅛ teaspoon red pepper flakes

16 pieces bacon, room temperature

1. Set the grill to low heat, and make a flat-bottom boat with aluminum foil large enough to hold 16 jalapeño halves, or use a grill mat.

2. Cut off the jalapeño stems, halve the peppers lengthwise, and scoop out the seeds with a knife or spoon.

3. In a small bowl, mash together the cream cheese, apricot preserves, and red pepper flakes until well incorporated. Using a butter knife, fill each of the jalapeño halves with the cream cheese mixture.

4. Starting at the stem end of the jalapeño, lay a piece of bacon lengthwise across the cream cheese down toward the pointed end, and then wrap bacon around the jalapeño all the way back to the stem end so the entire jalapeño is covered lengthwise. This keeps the cream cheese from bubbling out. Repeat with remaining peppers and bacon slices.

5. Place the jalapeños cream cheese–side down on the foil boat or mat, cook for 10 minutes, flip, and cook for an additional 10 minutes.

COOKING TIP

To cook these in the oven, preheat the oven to 375°F, and line a baking sheet with parchment paper. Add the firecrackers, cream cheese–side up, on the lined baking sheet, and cook for 20 to 30 minutes, until the bacon is crispy.

Per Serving (2 jalapeño halves): Calories: 163; Total Fat: 13g; Carbohydrates: 5g; Fiber: 1.5g; Net Carbs: 3.5g; Protein: 7g; Sugar Alcohols: 0g
Macros: Fat 72% Carbs 9% Protein 17%

Red, White, and Blue Parfaits

NUT-FREE, VEGETARIAN

Prep time: 15 minutes | **Servings:** 8

These parfaits are just perfect for a Fourth of July picnic, or anytime, for that matter. The presentation is so patriotic, and the sweet berries with the thick, creamy mousse taste delectable! For a picnic, I've got them served in 6- to 8-ounce plastic "to-go" glasses that are a little taller than needed so the lid doesn't mess up the topping. You could get fancier at home and put them in pretty parfait glasses or dessert dishes. If you can't find mascarpone cheese, cream cheese will do.

1½ cups heavy cream

½ cup confectioners' erythritol blend

½ teaspoon vanilla extract

8 ounces mascarpone cheese

1 cup raspberries

1 cup blueberries

1. In a medium bowl, combine the cream, confectioners' sweetener, and vanilla, and whip on high speed until soft peaks form, 45 to 60 seconds. Add the mascarpone cheese and whip on high speed, scraping down the sides of the bowl as you go, until it thickens and stiff peaks form, 30 to 45 seconds.

2. Line up 8 clear plastic cups or glasses, and drop an equal amount of raspberries in the bottom of each glass. Using a piping bag or resealable bag with the corner cut off, pipe about a ¼-cup layer of mousse on top of the raspberries in each glass. Place the blueberries evenly on top of the whipped cream in each glass, and then pipe a bit of whipped cream on top of the blueberries. Serve, or cover and refrigerate until ready to serve.

SPICE IT UP

This thick mousse is the perfect opportunity to use a piping bag with tips. Piping will add so much dimension to this dessert with great detail and a lovely effect. If you want a little crunch, feel free to sprinkle some chopped nuts on top.

Per Serving (1 parfait): Calories: 293; Total Fat: 30g; Carbohydrates: 13g; Fiber: 1.5g; Net Carbs: 4g; Protein: 4g; Sugar Alcohols: 7.5g
Macros: Fat 92% Carbs 5% Protein 5%

CHAPTER FIVE

Fall Festivities

Autumn is a feast for the senses, marked by colorful leaves, crisp air of cooler days, and the cozy aromas of apples, root vegetables, and hearty meals filling the home. We'll kick off this harvest season with a Rosh Hashanah celebration that includes all the trimmings. Next, we'll slink into Halloween with a variety of treats both creepy and sweet; then we head south of the border for a celebratory Día de los Muertos meal. Wrapping up this chapter's fall festivities is perhaps the most revered holiday of all—Thanksgiving—and since it's such a feast, it spills right over into the day after with a special pizza to use up all those leftovers.

Rosh Hashanah Celebration

Baba Ghanoush (page 88)
Slow Cooker Brisket (page 89)
Roasted Fall Vegetables (page 90)
Cinnamon Noodle Kugel (page 91)

Roasted Fall Vegetables, page 90

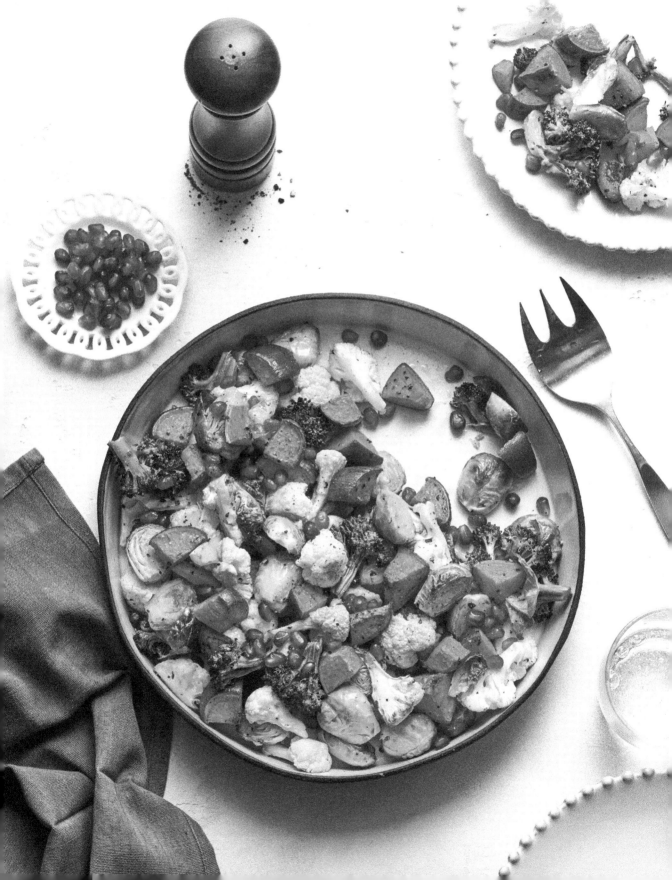

Baba Ghanoush

DAIRY-FREE, NUT-FREE, VEGAN

Prep time: 15 minutes | **Cook time:** 45 minutes | **Servings:** 8

I discovered baba ghanoush many years ago while traveling abroad and was smitten with how amazing and different it was—it's like the creamier keto cousin to hummus. Made with eggplant, tahini, and olive oil, it wasn't hard to keto-fy at all. I love to serve it as a dip with zucchini or cucumber slices or celery sticks at the start of any dinner party.

1 medium eggplant (1 to 1½ pounds)

¼ cup tahini

2 tablespoons freshly squeezed lemon juice

2 tablespoons olive oil, plus more for drizzling

1 teaspoon garlic powder

½ teaspoon salt

6 sliced kalamata olives, for garnish

Chopped parsley, for garnish

1. Preheat the oven to 350°F. Place aluminum foil on the middle rack, place the eggplant on the aluminum foil, and bake for 45 to 60 minutes, or until the eggplant is fork-tender and the skin very wrinkly.

2. Remove from the oven and cut the eggplant lengthwise. Scoop out the insides, discarding the skins, drain the liquid, and place the insides in a food processor or blender.

3. Add the tahini, lemon juice, olive oil, garlic powder, and salt to the food processor, and blend into a paste for 2 minutes.

4. Transfer to a serving bowl or plate, and garnish with the olives, parsley, and a drizzle of olive oil.

PAIR IT
Serve this yummy dish with the crackers or "scoops" from the Sriracha Artichoke Bites (page 136).

Per Serving (2 tablespoons): Calories: 86; Total Fat: 6.5g; Carbohydrates: 6.5g; Fiber: 2.5g; Net Carbs: 4g; Protein: 2g; Sugar Alcohols: 0g
Macros: Fat 68% Carbs 19% Protein 9%

Slow Cooker Brisket

DAIRY-FREE, NUT-FREE

Prep time: 15 minutes | **Cook time:** 8 hours | **Servings:** 8

Brisket is a traditional main dish for the Jewish high holidays, but it's also a great choice for any occasion, especially when you have a lot of people to feed. During the holidays, my ovens are usually in full use, so the slow cooker comes in handy and takes up very little counter space. Fat is the key for a tasty brisket, so I recommend choosing a cut of meat with a flat shape and lots of fat. First or second cut (like you find at the grocery store) will work great. When possible, I'll splurge for the higher-quality meat, organic and hormone-free. Don't trim off the fat, and cook the meat low and slow for the most flavorful and fork-tender brisket ever!

1 teaspoon garlic powder

1 teaspoon Lawry's seasoned salt

1 teaspoon minced onion

½ teaspoon freshly ground black pepper

4- to 6-pound beef brisket

3 to 4 cups beef broth or bone broth

1. In a small bowl, mix the garlic powder, seasoned salt, minced onion, and pepper. Spread it on all sides of the meat. Place the meat into the slow cooker. If the brisket is too big, cut it to fit.

2. Pour the broth over the meat, cover, and cook for 8 hours on low. Serve topped with its own juice.

PREP TIP

If you have time, season the brisket, cover in plastic wrap, and refrigerate overnight before cooking.

Per Serving: Calories: 538; Total Fat: 36g; Carbohydrates: 1g; Fiber: 0g; Net Carbs: 1g; Protein: 50g; Sugar Alcohols: 0g
Macros: Fat 60% Carbs 1% Protein 37%

Roasted Fall Vegetables

DAIRY-FREE, NUT-FREE, VEGAN

Prep time: 10 minutes | **Cook time:** 1 hour | **Servings:** 8

Roasted vegetables are so good, but a mixture of sweet roasted veggies with tart pomegranate seeds is like an explosion of fall flavor in your mouth. I added some sweet potato to this recipe, which makes it a little more carby, so you could leave that out if you're really tracking, but the flavor it adds is worth it if you can spare the carbs.

1 small head cauliflower, cut into small florets (about 2 cups)

1 small sweet potato, cut into ½-inch cubes

½ pound Brussels sprouts (about 2 cups), bottoms cut, wilted leaves removed, and halved

½ pound broccoli, cut into small florets (about 2 cups)

3 tablespoons olive oil, divided

1 teaspoon garlic powder

1 teaspoon salt

½ teaspoon freshly ground black pepper

½ cup pomegranate seeds

1. Preheat the oven to 425°F, and line two baking sheets with parchment paper.

2. In a gallon resealable bag, combine half of each of the vegetables: cauliflower, sweet potato, Brussels sprouts, and broccoli. Add 1 tablespoon of olive oil, seal, and massage and turn the bag until well coated. Spread evenly on baking tray and season with half the garlic powder, salt, and pepper. Bake for 30 to 40 minutes, rotating the baking sheet halfway through. Repeat with the remaining vegetables, garlic powder, salt, and pepper on the second baking sheet.

3. Transfer the roasted vegetables to a large serving bowl. Drizzle the vegetables with the remaining tablespoon of oil and half the pomegranate seeds, and gently toss. Sprinkle the remaining seeds on top and serve.

Per Serving: Calories: 95; Total Fat: 5.5g; Carbohydrates: 10.5g; Fiber: 3.5g; Net Carbs: 7g; Protein: 3g; Sugar Alcohols: 0g
Macros: Fat 52% Carbs 29% Protein 13%

Cinnamon Noodle Kugel

VEGETARIAN

Prep time: 20 minutes | **Cook time:** 1 hour 30 minutes | **Servings:** 10

There are many types of kugel—it can be made with potatoes or noodles; it can be savory or sweet. Apple cinnamon has to be my favorite, though! I substituted spaghetti squash for the noodles, and jicama for the apple. This dish just comes together so easily!

Oil or nonstick cooking spray, for greasing

2½- to 3-pound spaghetti squash (about 1 medium squash)

1 tablespoon olive oil

1 small jicama, peeled and grated

4 large eggs

1 cup granulated erythritol blend

4 ounces (½ brick) cream cheese

½ teaspoon vanilla extract

1 teaspoon cinnamon

1 teaspoon apple pie spice

½ cup almond flour

¼ cup brown erythritol blend

2 tablespoons melted butter

½ teaspoon cinnamon

1. Preheat the oven to 425°F, line a baking sheet with parchment paper, and lightly grease an 8-inch square baking dish.

2. Cut the spaghetti squash in half lengthwise, and scoop out the seeds and strings. Drizzle with olive oil and place cut-side down on the lined baking sheet. Bake for 30 minutes, turn over, and cook another 5 minutes. Remove from the oven, set aside to cool, and reduce the oven temperature to 350°F.

3. Using a fork, rake the squash strands into a small colander or cheesecloth, and squeeze out the excess water. Place in a medium bowl, and add the grated jicama.

4. In a blender, combine the eggs, sweetener, cream cheese, vanilla, cinnamon, and apple pie spice. Pulse 2 or 3 times until blended, pour over the spaghetti squash and jicama, mix, and pour into the prepared baking dish.

5. In a small bowl, stir together the almond flour, brown sweetener, butter, and cinnamon. Sprinkle over the top of the dish, cover with aluminum foil, bake for 40 minutes, remove the foil, and bake another 15 minutes, or until the topping is golden brown. Let sit for 5 to 10 minutes, and serve.

Per Serving: Calories: 179; Total Fat: 13g; Carbohydrates: 35g; Fiber: 4g; Net Carbs: 7g; Protein: 5g; Sugar Alcohols: 24g
Macros: Fat 65% Carbs 16% Protein 11%

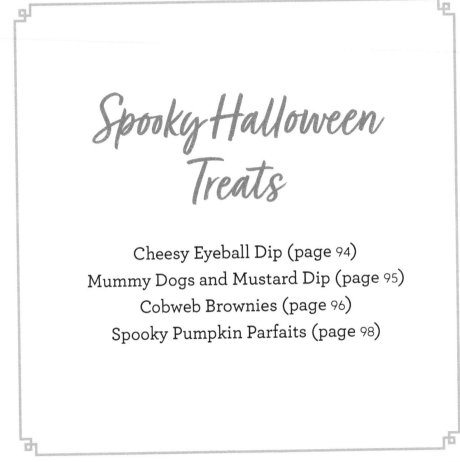

Spooky Halloween Treats

Cobweb Brownies, page 96

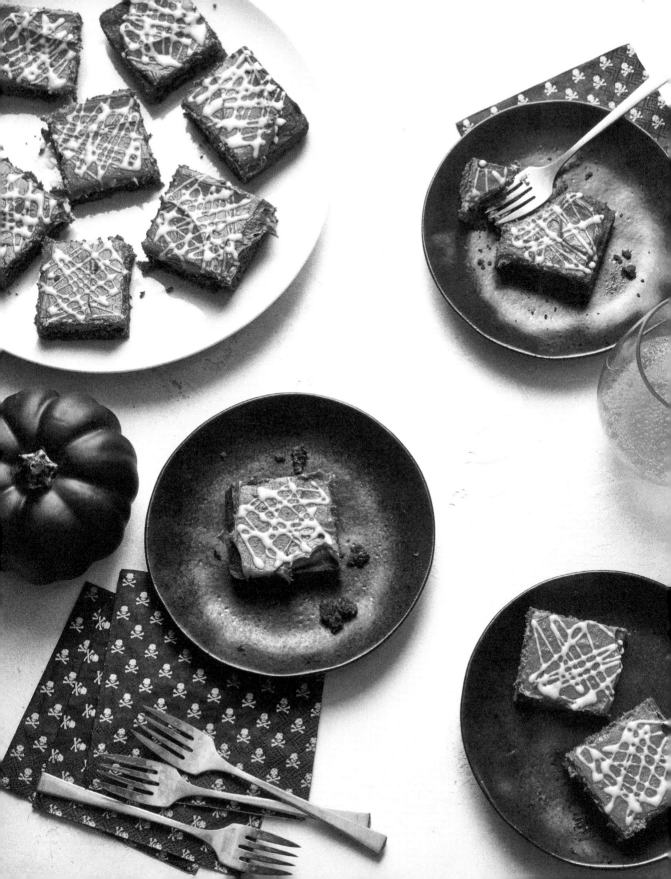

Cheesy Eyeball Dip

NUT-FREE, VEGETARIAN

Prep time: 15 minutes, plus 2 hours to chill | **Servings:** 10

Creepy bloodshot eyeballs are perfect for Halloween, and this cheese ball makes an authentic-looking eyeball that tastes delicious. To get some creative courage for piping the bloodshot eyes, google "bloodshot Halloween eyes," and you'll get lots of examples. There's no way to get it wrong—just have fun with it! It's also great to make ahead of time and then add the decorations when you're ready to serve.

16 ounces (2 bricks) cream cheese, room temperature

1 (1-ounce) packet ranch dressing mix

1 cup shredded white cheddar cheese

1 teaspoon minced garlic

1 spinach leaf, cut in a circle for the eye (1 to 2 inches in diameter)

1 black olive, cut in half for the pupil

¼ cup sriracha sauce or sugar-free ketchup for veins on eyeballs

10 celery stalks, cut in thirds

1. In a large bowl, mix together the cream cheese and ranch seasoning. Add the white cheddar and minced garlic, mix well, and form into a ball. Cover and refrigerate for at least 2 hours.

2. Remove from the refrigerator and place the round spinach cutout in the center on top of the cheese ball. Set the black olive in the center of the spinach, pressing in to secure. Using a piping bag or resealable bag with the very tip of one corner cut off, pipe the sriracha or ketchup in the shape of red veins on the cheese ball, branching off to make them look spooky. Serve with celery sticks for dipping.

PAIR IT
This dip would also be great with the crackers made from the "scoops" recipe on page 136.

Per Serving (3 pieces celery and ⅒ of the dip): Calories: 219; Total Fat: 19g; Carbohydrates: 7g; Fiber: 0.5g; Net Carbs: 6.5g; Protein: 6g; Sugar Alcohols: 0g
Macros: Fat 78% Carbs 12% Protein 11%

Mummy Dogs and Mustard Dip

Prep time: 20 minutes | **Cook time:** 20 minutes | **Hot dogs:** 10

I've made these cute mummy hot dogs for as long as I can remember. It's fun to make their eyes go in different directions, which gives them character. It's also something you can do with the kiddos—they'll love it!

¾ cup grated mozzarella cheese

1 ounce (2 tablespoons) cream cheese

¼ cup almond flour

1 tablespoon flaxseed meal

⅛ teaspoon salt

10 hot dogs

½ cup mayonnaise, plus 2 tablespoons for piping eyes

20 peppercorns

3 tablespoons yellow mustard

2 tablespoons sriracha sauce (optional)

1. Preheat the oven to 350°F, and line a baking sheet with parchment paper.

2. In a microwave-safe bowl, melt the mozzarella cheese and cream cheese in the microwave in 20-second increments, until the mozzarella is melted and smooth. Remove from the microwave and mix in the almond flour, flaxseed, and salt, and work into a ball of dough (it will be greasy).

3. Spread a piece of parchment paper on the counter, and place the dough on top. Place another parchment paper on top, and with a rolling pin or side of a drinking glass, roll the dough very thin, 1/16 to 1/8 inch thick. Using a pizza cutter or knife, cut strips about ¼ inch wide. Wrap one or two strips of dough around each hot dog to look like bandages. At the top of each hot dog, about ½ inch down, leave a space uncovered for the eyes.

4. Place the wrapped hot dogs on the baking tray and bake for 15 to 20 minutes, or until golden brown, rotating the hot dogs halfway through.

5. Let the hot dogs cool. Add 2 tablespoons of mayonnaise to a resealable bag, and clip the very end of the bag. Pipe two white dots at the top of the hot dog for eyes, and place a peppercorn in the center of each dot.

6. In a small bowl, mix together ½ cup of mayonnaise, the mustard, and the sriracha (if using), and serve as dip with the hot dogs.

Per Serving (1 hot dog): Calories: 256; Total Fat: 23g; Carbohydrates: 1g; Fiber: 0.5g; Net Carbs: 0.5g; Protein: 10g; Sugar Alcohols: 0g
Macros: Fat 81% Carbs 1% Protein 16%

Cobweb Brownies

VEGETARIAN

Prep time: 10 minutes | **Cook time:** 20 minutes | **Brownies:** 16

The first thing I ever baked from scratch was brownies. I was only seven or eight at the time, but I became a real baker, and every weekend I would whip up a batch to share with the neighbors or pack in my lunchbox to take to school. When I started keto, my brownie baking days came to an abrupt halt until I figured out how to make these delicious morsels once again. I've got to say, they're pretty dang good, but don't overlook the pepper that's called for—trust me and put it in there. And whether you enjoy them cake-like, as I do, or fudgy, these brownies will make you smile! I like Lily's Dark Chocolate Chips for this recipe, but you can use any sugar-free chips.

FOR THE BROWNIES

½ cup (1 stick) butter, room temperature (not melted)

6 tablespoons unsweetened cocoa powder

3 large eggs for cake-like brownies or 2 eggs for fudgy

1 teaspoon vanilla extract

1½ cups almond flour

1 cup confectioners' erythritol blend

1 teaspoon baking powder

¼ teaspoon freshly ground black pepper

¼ cup sugar-free chocolate chips

FOR THE CHOCOLATE ICING

2 cups confectioners' erythritol blend

¼ cup unsweetened cocoa powder

¼ cup (½ stick) butter, softened

8 teaspoons boiling water

1 teaspoon vanilla extract

FOR THE COBWEB DRIZZLE

½ cup confectioners' erythritol blend

2 teaspoons water or sugar-free almond milk

1. Preheat the oven to 350°F, and line an 8-inch square baking dish with parchment paper hanging a bit over the edges so you can grip it later.

2. **To make the brownies:** In a medium bowl or bowl of a stand mixer, whip the butter until creamy. Beat in the cocoa powder, eggs, and vanilla.

3. In a small bowl, stir together the almond flour, confectioners' sweetener, baking powder, and pepper, and add to the chocolate mixture. Stir until incorporated, fold in the chocolate chips, and pour into the pan.

4. Bake for 20 to 23 minutes, turning the pan halfway through for even baking. Test for doneness at 20 minutes by inserting a knife in the brownies. If the knife comes out clean, they're done. Allow to completely cool on the counter.

5. **To make the chocolate icing:** In a medium bowl, mix together the confectioners' sweetener and cocoa. Add the butter, boiling water, and vanilla, and mix with a hand mixer for 45 seconds to a minute. Spread the icing over the cool brownies. Carefully lift the parchment paper and brownies out of the pan, place on the counter, and cut into 16 servings.

6. **To make the cobweb drizzle:** In a small bowl, mix the confectioners' sweetener and water, and spoon into a piping bag or resealable bag with the corner snipped. Quickly darting back and forth and side to side over the brownies, pipe strands in all directions to look like spiderwebs across the top.

SPICE IT UP
If you're a nut lover, add ¼ cup of chopped pecans or walnuts to the batter before cooking, or sprinkle them across the top of the icing for decoration.

Per Serving (1 brownie): Calories: 164; Total Fat: 15g; Carbohydrates: 28g; Fiber: 2.5g; Net Carbs: 3g; Protein: 4g; Sugar Alcohols: 22.5g
Macros: Fat 82% Carbs 7% Protein 10%

Spooky Pumpkin Parfaits

NUT-FREE, VEGETARIAN

Prep time: 30 minutes | **Parfaits:** 10

What's Halloween without a pumpkin dessert? Pumpkin mousse is delicious on its own, but the addition of chocolate and vanilla makes this parfait a party in your mouth! So rich and full of flavor, just a little goes a long way—in fact, I like to layer mine in shot glasses, but you could also layer them in small parfait glasses. Just make sure your glass is wide enough to fit a small spoon. I used three piping bags for this recipe. You don't have to use a tip; you can just cut off the bottom of the bag and pipe. There's no wrong way to do this. Just lean into it and have fun!

2 cups heavy cream, divided

1½ cups confectioners' erythritol blend

12 ounces mascarpone or cream cheese, room temperature

1 teaspoon vanilla extract

¾ cup 100 percent pure pumpkin, canned, unsweetened

¼ teaspoon pumpkin pie spice

3 tablespoons cocoa powder, unsweetened

1. In a large bowl using a hand mixer, whip 1½ cups of heavy cream and confectioners' sweetener on high for 90 seconds. Cube the mascarpone, add it to the whipped cream along with the vanilla, and whip on high for another 45 seconds, until the mixture begins to thicken.

2. Transfer three-quarters of the mixture to another bowl. To the remaining mixture, add the pumpkin and pumpkin pie spice. Beat the ingredients on high for 30 to 45 seconds. Transfer the pumpkin mixture to a piping bag, rinse the bowl and beaters, and add half the vanilla mousse back into the bowl.

3. Add the cocoa powder and remaining ½ cup of heavy cream, and beat the ingredients for 1 minute, starting on low so the cocoa doesn't blow out of the bowl. Transfer the mixture to a piping bag.

4. Transfer the remaining vanilla mousse to a piping bag and set aside.

5. Starting with the chocolate mousse bag, pipe evenly among the glasses, tap the glasses on the counter to smooth it out, and then pipe the vanilla on top. Shake the glass again to even it out, pipe the pumpkin on top of the vanilla, and serve.

SPICE IT UP

Perch some small plastic spiders on top for an extra spooky effect!

Per Serving (1 parfait): Calories: 320; Total Fat: 33g; Carbohydrates: 20.5g; Fiber: 1g; Net Carbs: 2.5g; Protein: 4g; Sugar Alcohols: 17g
Macros: Fat 93% Carbs 3% Protein 5%

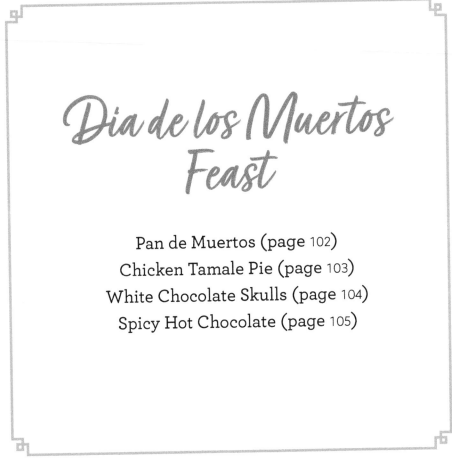

Dia de los Muertos Feast

Pan de Muertos (page 102)
Chicken Tamale Pie (page 103)
White Chocolate Skulls (page 104)
Spicy Hot Chocolate (page 105)

Chicken Tamale Pie, page 103

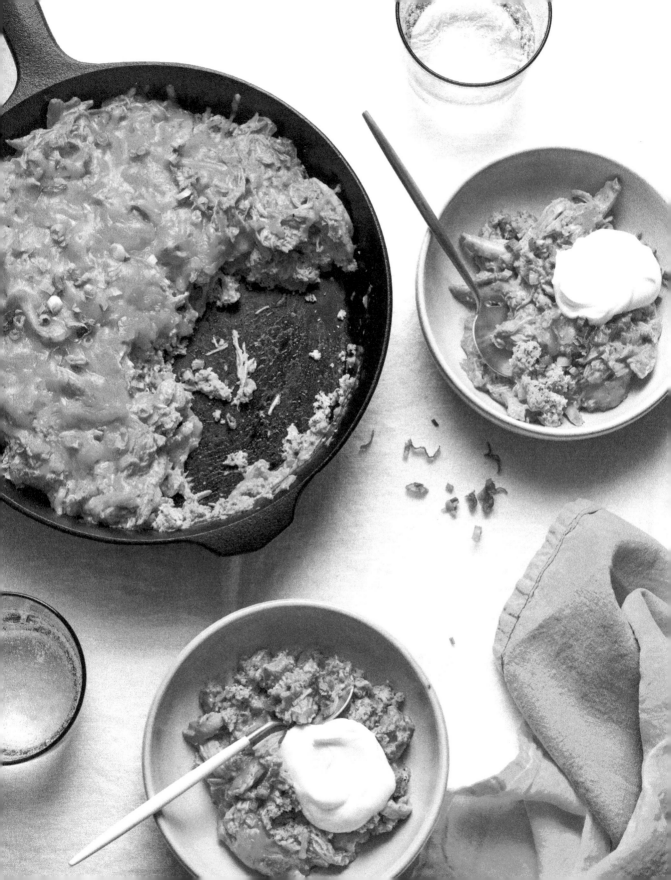

Pan de Muertos

VEGETARIAN

Prep time: 5 minutes, plus 30 minutes to chill | **Cook time:** 20 minutes | **Rolls:** 4

Pan de Muertos, or "Bread of the Dead," is a traditional sweet bread served during Día de los Muertos as an offering for departed loved ones. I was so excited to get this recipe just right because on the occasions I've had it, it was absolutely delicious.

1 cup almond flour

½ cup golden flaxseed meal (or any color)

1 teaspoon baking powder

⅛ teaspoon salt

¼ cup (½ stick) butter, room temperature or softened, divided

2 tablespoons cream cheese, room temperature or softened

2 large eggs, divided

2 teaspoons orange zest

½ teaspoon orange extract

1 teaspoon anise seeds

2 teaspoons granulated erythritol blend

1. In a medium bowl, combine the flour, flaxseed, baking powder, and salt, and stir together. Add 3 tablespoons of butter, cream cheese, 1 egg, orange zest, orange extract, and anise seeds, and mix together (it will be sticky). Wrap the dough in plastic wrap, and refrigerate for at least 30 minutes or longer if possible.

2. Preheat the oven to 325°F, and line a baking sheet with parchment paper.

3. Divide the dough in quarters. Pinch a ½-inch piece off each one, roll the bigger portions in a ball, pat them down just a bit, and place on the lined baking sheet. Take a small piece off the ½-inch piece, and roll into a ball. Roll the remaining small piece of dough into a snake, cut it in two, and place like a cross over the roll. Make a dent in the middle of the cross and add the ball.

4. Beat the remaining egg and brush it over each roll, and then bake for 20 minutes.

5. Allow the rolls to cool for a few minutes, and then melt the remaining tablespoon of butter and brush across the tops. Sprinkle the sweetener evenly over the top and sides of each one before serving.

Per Serving (1 roll): Calories: 349; Total Fat: 31g; Carbohydrates: 10.5g; Fiber: 6g; Net Carbs: 2.5g; Protein: 11g; Sugar Alcohols: 2g
Macros: Fat 80% Carbs 3% Protein 13%

Chicken Tamale Pie

NUT-FREE

Prep time: 15 minutes | **Cook time:** 35 minutes | **Servings:** 8

This is such an easy and flavorful recipe, and it tastes pretty close to tamales without all the work. You could also use shredded brisket or beef—it's all good! Feel free to spice this up with some cayenne or chili powder as well.

FOR THE MUFFINS
Nonstick cooking spray
1 cup coconut flour
¼ cup flaxseed meal
½ teaspoon
  baking powder
½ teaspoon garlic powder
4 large eggs
¼ cup heavy cream
¼ cup buttermilk

FOR THE CHICKEN
1½ pounds
  shredded chicken
1 (10-ounce) can red
  enchilada sauce (mild,
  medium, or hot to taste)
4 ounces (½ brick)
  cream cheese
1 (4-ounce) can chopped
  green chiles

¼ cup heavy cream
1 teaspoon taco seasoning
1 cup grated
  cheddar cheese
2 scallions, chopped,
  for garnish

1. **To make the muffins:** Preheat the oven to 350°F, and grease 8 holes of a standard muffin pan with nonstick cooking spray.

2. In a medium bowl, stir together the flour, flaxseed, baking powder, and garlic powder.

3. In a small bowl, whisk together the eggs, cream, and buttermilk. Pour the egg mixture into the flour mixture, and stir together. Spoon evenly into 8 muffin holes, and bake for 25 to 30 minutes. If the tops get too brown while cooking, cover loosely with aluminum foil.

4. Leaving the oven on, remove the muffins, chop them up, and spread on the bottom of a medium cast-iron skillet or 1½-quart baking dish.

5. **To make the chicken:** In a large skillet over medium heat, combine the chicken, enchilada sauce, cream cheese, green chiles, cream, and taco seasoning. Cook until heated through. Pour over the muffins, top evenly with the cheddar cheese, and return to the oven for about 5 minutes to melt the cheese. Garnish with the scallions, and serve.

Per Serving: Calories: 423; Total Fat: 28g; Carbohydrates: 15g; Fiber: 7.5g; Net Carbs: 7.5g; Protein: 29g; Sugar Alcohols: 0g
Macros: Fat 60% Carbs 7% Protein 27%

White Chocolate Skulls

DAIRY-FREE, NUT-FREE, VEGAN

Prep time: 5 minutes, plus 30 minutes to chill | **Cook time:** 5 minutes | **Skulls:** 3 (2-ounce)

In Mexico, sugar skulls represent a departed soul. They have big, happy smiles made from colorful icing and are a huge part of the Día de los Muertos ("Day of the Dead") holiday. I took a little creative freedom and went the white chocolate route. I used a sugar skull mold, but I provide instructions for drawing and piping your own so you don't need a specialty mold. If you do want to use a mold, check the hobby stores or look on Amazon. You can order larger individual molds or a sheet of smaller ones—it's up to you, but adjust the nutritional info accordingly.

1 (7-ounce) bag sugar-free white chocolate chips (see tip)

Gel colors, for decorating

1. Place a glass or metal bowl on top of a small pan with about 2 inches of water in the bottom on medium heat. Place the white chocolate in the bowl, and as the water underneath begins to boil, turn off the heat and continue to stir until the chocolate is melted. If using a mold, spoon the melted chocolate into your mold.

2. Alternatively, using a pencil, trace or draw three skulls about 3 inches in diameter on wax paper. Put some melted chocolate in a piping bag or resealable bag and cut a tiny bit off the corner, and pipe along your traced line. Place in the refrigerator for a minute (just long enough to harden up), and then remove and pipe more chocolate to fill in the skull.

3. Refrigerate the skull(s) for 30 minutes or until completely hardened. Remove from the mold or peel off the wax paper, and decorate as you like using small paintbrushes or cotton swabs and the gel colors.

PREP TIP
I used ChocZero's sugar-free white chocolate chips, but any sugar-free white chocolate will work. Paint your skulls in thin layers so the gels will have a chance to dry as you go along.

Per Serving (1 skull): Calories: 369; Total Fat: 24g; Carbohydrates: 33g; Fiber: 28g; Net Carbs: 5g; Protein: 5g; Sugar Alcohols: 0g
Macros: Fat 59% Carbs 5% Protein 5%

Spicy Hot Chocolate

DAIRY-FREE, VEGAN

Prep time: 10 minutes | **Servings:** 4

This spicy hot chocolate is like the sexier cousin of the hot chocolate I grew up with. It's thick and cozy but not too sweet, and it's full of rich chocolaty flavor that makes it feel like more of a dessert than a drink. The nutmeg and cinnamon add extra flavor, and a kick of cayenne pepper takes the chocolate to a whole new level. Of course, it's perfect on a cold night, but I also love to load it in a blender with ice and serve it frozen on a summer day.

- 1 (13.66-ounce) can unsweetened coconut cream
- 1½ cups sugar-free vanilla almond milk
- 4 tablespoons unsweetened cocoa powder
- 3 tablespoons brown erythritol blend
- 1 teaspoon cinnamon, plus more for sprinkling on top
- 1 teaspoon vanilla extract
- ⅛ teaspoon nutmeg
- ⅛ teaspoon cayenne pepper

1. In a small saucepan over low heat, combine the coconut cream, almond milk, cocoa powder, brown sweetener, cinnamon, vanilla, nutmeg, and cayenne pepper.

2. Whisk occasionally until heated through.

3. Pour into glasses, and top with a sprinkle of cinnamon.

SPICE IT UP

This drink doesn't need much more, but you could spice it up with a little more cayenne or even spike it with a shot of tequila.

Per Serving: Calories: 216; Total Fat: 21g; Carbohydrates: 15g; Fiber: 2.5g; Net Carbs: 3.5g; Protein: 1g; Sugar Alcohols: 9g
Macros: Fat 88% Carbs 6% Protein 2%

Thanksgiving Dinner (and the Day After)

Roast Turkey (page 108)

Green Bean Casserole (page 109)

"Cornbread" Sausage Dressing (page 110)

Cheesy Mashed Cauliflower (page 112)

Cranberry Sauce (page 113)

Pumpkin Pie (page 114)

Thanksgiving Leftovers Pizza (page 116)

Roast Turkey, page 108

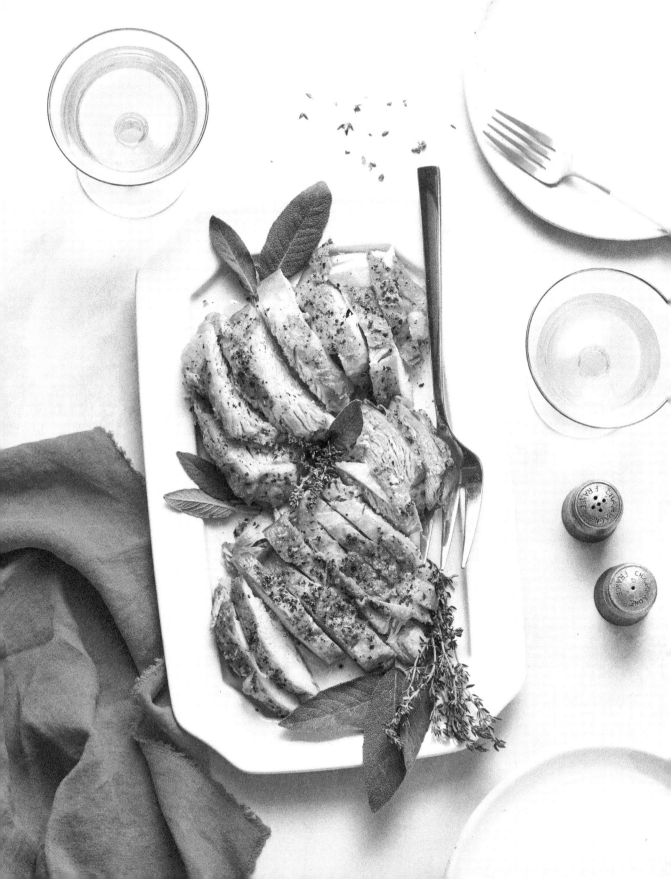

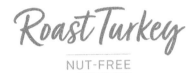

Roast Turkey

NUT-FREE

Prep time: 15 minutes | **Cook time:** 3 hours | **Servings:** 8

Since turkey is the main centerpiece for Thanksgiving, I've tried many different versions to see what worked best. The easiest way, I found, was to let it dry out overnight and then roast it Thanksgiving morning. We always eat in the early afternoon, so the turkey goes in around 8:30 a.m., and by noon, it's showtime. I always choose a fresh turkey at the store a few days in advance or order ahead of time from the butcher. If you do buy a frozen turkey, allow at least 2 days for it to thaw in the refrigerator.

10- to 12-pound turkey (with no added ingredients)

1 cup (2 sticks) butter

2 tablespoons chopped thyme

2 tablespoons chopped sage

1 teaspoon salt

1 teaspoon freshly ground black pepper

1. The night before cooking, remove the packaging and allow the turkey to sit uncovered in the refrigerator overnight to dry out. In the morning, remove the neck, giblets, and liver from the cavity, and discard.

2. Preheat the oven to 350°F, and place a rack in a roasting pan. Melt the butter in the microwave, and mix with the thyme and sage. Rub half the mixture all over the skin of the bird, lifting the skin to rub as much on the underside of the skin as possible. Season all over with the salt and pepper. Place on the roasting rack, breast-side up, cover with aluminum foil, and roast for 2 hours (add 15 minutes per pound for a larger turkey).

3. Remove the foil, increase the oven temperature to 425°F, baste with the remaining butter, and place back in the oven for another hour. Allow to rest for 30 minutes before carving.

COOKING TIP

I know a lot of folks like to baste the turkey every 10 or 15 minutes, but opening and closing the oven door increases the possibility of losing heat, so I don't recommend it. If you cover it in the butter and seasonings as directed, you should be fine.

Per Serving: Calories: 447; Total Fat: 21g; Carbohydrates: 0g; Fiber: 0g; Net Carbs: 0g; Protein: 66g; Sugar Alcohols: 0g
Macros: Fat 42% Carbs 0% Protein 59%

Green Bean Casserole

Prep time: 10 minutes | **Cook time:** 25 minutes | **Servings:** 8

Green beans surrounded by creamy mushroom sauce and topped with French's Crispy Fried Onions is a Thanksgiving classic. This keto version tastes pretty dang close to the original; I replaced the fried onions with a crispy bacon topping that is marvelous.

Oil or nonstick cooking spray, for greasing

6 slices bacon

3 ounces shiitake mushrooms, chopped into ¼-inch cubes (about 1 cup)

½ cup chopped white onion

1 tablespoon soy sauce

1 teaspoon garlic powder

1 teaspoon freshly ground black pepper

½ teaspoon salt

1 cup beef bone broth

½ cup heavy cream

½ teaspoon xanthan gum

2 (14½-ounce) cans green beans, drained; 1½ pounds fresh, blanched; or 16 to 20 ounces frozen, thawed

½ cup almond flour

2 tablespoons melted butter

1. Preheat the oven to 350°F. Grease a baking dish, and set it aside.

2. In a medium skillet over medium heat, fry the bacon until crisp. Remove and set aside, reserving the grease in the pan. Chop the bacon when cool.

3. To the pan with the bacon grease, add the mushrooms, onion, soy sauce, garlic powder, pepper, and salt, and stir continuously for 4 to 6 minutes, until tender. Add the bone broth and heavy cream, and stir until bubbles appear. Add the xanthan gum, reduce heat, and stir for another 3 or 4 minutes as it thickens. Add the green beans, mix well, and pour into the prepared baking dish.

4. In a small bowl, stir together the chopped bacon, almond flour, and melted butter. Sprinkle over the top of the green bean casserole. Bake for 10 to 15 minutes, or until the topping is browned. Serve warm.

COOKING TIP

If you use fresh green beans in this recipe, you will need to blanch them first. Boil them for 5 minutes, then drop them in an ice water bath to cool quickly. Drain and use in the recipe.

Per Serving: Calories: 246; Total Fat: 22g; Carbohydrates: 9g; Fiber: 3.5g; Net Carbs: 5.5g; Protein: 7g; Sugar Alcohols: 0g
Macros: Fat 80% Carbs 9% Protein 11%

"Cornbread" Sausage Dressing

NUT-FREE

Prep time: 15 minutes | **Cook time:** 1 hour 20 minutes | **Servings:** 10

Growing up, I would watch my mother lay the bread and cornbread out on the counter with just a kitchen towel covering them so they could dry out overnight. The next morning, she would mix up all the ingredients and make the most incredible dressing ever! This keto-friendly version is so much like the original in both taste and texture. I love to serve it for Thanksgiving but enjoy it many other days as well.

Oil or nonstick cooking spray, for greasing

4 large eggs

¼ cup heavy cream

¼ cup buttermilk

1 tablespoon avocado oil or olive oil

1 cup coconut flour

¼ cup flaxseed meal

½ teaspoon baking powder

2 tablespoons granulated erythritol blend

16 ounces breakfast sausage

½ chopped white onion

4 celery stalks, chopped

2 cups beef bone broth

1. Preheat the oven to 350°F, and grease 8 holes of a standard muffin pan and a medium baking dish. Line a baking sheet with parchment paper.

2. In a medium bowl, whisk together the eggs, heavy cream, buttermilk, and oil.

3. In a small bowl, stir together the flour, flaxseed, baking powder, and sweetener. Use the back of a spoon to mash out any lumps. Pour the flour mixture into the egg mixture, mixing to blend. Spoon the mixture evenly into the prepared muffin pan.

4. Bake for 25 to 30 minutes. If the tops get too brown, cover loosely with aluminum foil.

5. Reduce the oven temperature to 300°F. When cool enough to handle, remove the muffins from the pan, and chop into ½-inch cubes. Spread evenly on the lined baking sheet, and put back in the oven for 20 minutes.

6. Meanwhile, in a medium skillet over medium heat, cook the sausage. When cooked through, add the onion and celery; cook, stirring occasionally, for another 3 to 5 minutes; and pour into the prepared baking dish.

7. Add the "cornbread" to the sausage mixture, and fold together. Pour the bone broth over the mixture, cover with foil, and bake for 30 minutes. Uncover and cook another 10 minutes. Serve warm.

COOKING TIP
If the dressing looks too dry, add some additional bone broth, stir, and put back in the oven for a few minutes.

Per Serving: Calories: 287; Total Fat: 21g; Carbohydrates: 12g; Fiber: 6g; Net Carbs: 3.5g; Protein: 14g; Sugar Alcohols: 2.5g
Macros: Fat 66% Carbs 5% Protein 20%

Cheesy Mashed Cauliflower

NUT-FREE, VEGETARIAN

Prep time: 10 minutes | **Cook time:** 30 minutes | **Servings:** 8

There's nothing more "comfort food" than mashed potatoes, but my recipe for cheesy mashed cauliflower comes pretty dang close! It's rich and creamy and oh so cheesy. It's also the perfect side for any holiday or everyday meal. I think one of the biggest challenges folks have with turning cauliflower into potato look-alikes is that they steam their cauliflower, making the outcome very watery. I like to roast my cauliflower, which dries it out and makes the most incredible version ever!

2 cauliflower heads, cut into florets (about 16 cups)

2 tablespoons olive oil

2 tablespoons butter

4 garlic cloves, minced

½ cup buttermilk, plus more if needed

1 teaspoon garlic powder

1 teaspoon salt

½ teaspoon freshly ground black pepper

½ cup grated Parmesan cheese

½ cup mascarpone cheese

1. Preheat the oven to 450°F, and line a baking sheet with parchment paper.

2. In a gallon resealable bag, add the cauliflower and olive oil, seal, and massage and turn to coat. Spread the cauliflower evenly on the lined baking sheet, and roast for 25 to 30 minutes, until fork-tender.

3. In a large pan over medium heat, melt the butter. Add the garlic and sauté for 30 to 45 seconds; then remove from heat, add the cauliflower, and stir. Add the buttermilk, garlic powder, salt, and pepper. Using an immersion blender, blend to desired consistency. Alternatively, pour the cauliflower into a food processor or blender and blend (being careful not to splatter hot liquid), or mash with a potato masher.

4. Stir in the Parmesan and mascarpone. If it's too thick, add a little more buttermilk. Transfer to a bowl and serve.

Per Serving: Calories: 260; Total Fat: 22g; Carbohydrates: 13g; Fiber: 4.5g; Net Carbs: 8.5g; Protein: 8g; Sugar Alcohols: 0g
Macros: Fat 76% Carbs 13% Protein 12%

Cranberry Sauce

DAIRY-FREE, NUT-FREE, VEGAN

Prep time: 5 minutes | **Cook time:** 15 minutes | **Servings:** 10

Growing up, we always had the cranberry sauce right out of the can. It was my job to grab the can opener and open it, along with the black olives. It's funny looking back on it because in other areas we were pretty fancy, but not with cranberry sauce. The first time I had the real thing, I was so excited and couldn't imagine why we hadn't had the homemade stuff all along, especially when I discovered how easy it was to make. Fortunately, it was easy to keto-fy as well and just as good.

12 ounces fresh cranberries, or frozen, thawed

1¼ cups water
1 cup confectioners' erythritol blend

2 tablespoons brown erythritol blend
1 teaspoon cinnamon

1. In a medium saucepan over medium heat, combine the cranberries, water, confectioners' sweetener, brown sweetener, and cinnamon. Bring to a boil, stirring occasionally.

2. Reduce heat to a simmer, and stir until the cranberry skins begin to burst.

3. Remove from heat, and use a fork to mash the cranberries to desired consistency. Refrigerate until ready to serve.

SPICE IT UP
If you want a little heat with your cranberry sauce, add some pepper flakes or cayenne pepper. Don't make that face—it's a really good complement to the sweetness!

Per Serving (¼ cup): Calories: 16; Total Fat: 0g; Carbohydrates: 19g; Fiber: 1.5g; Net Carbs: 3g; Protein: 0g; Sugar Alcohols: 14.5g
Macros: Fat 0% Carbs 75% Protein 0%

Pumpkin Pie

VEGETARIAN

Prep time: 20 minutes | **Cook time:** 1 hour, plus 1 hour to cool in the oven | **Servings:** 8

I can't have holidays without pumpkin pie, especially Thanksgiving, but the other holidays are worthy of it as well. I remember my mother always bought two pumpkin pies, along with the ubiquitous tub of Cool Whip to dollop on top. One was to share with guests or take to a family gathering; the other was for us to have with leftovers. As I got older, I learned to make this wonderful dessert from scratch, and when I started keto, it was one of the first desserts I keto-fied.

FOR THE DOUGH

¾ cup coconut flour

¼ cup ground pecans

2 tablespoons granulated erythritol blend

⅛ teaspoon salt

6 tablespoons melted butter

FOR THE FILLING

3 large eggs

1 (15-ounce) can 100 percent pure pumpkin, unsweetened

1 cup confectioners' erythritol blend

1 cup heavy cream

1 teaspoon pumpkin pie spice

¼ teaspoon finely ground black pepper

1 teaspoon vanilla extract

FOR THE SUGAR-FREE WHIPPED CREAM

1 cup heavy cream

1 tablespoon confectioners' erythritol blend

½ teaspoon vanilla extract

1. Preheat the oven to 350°F.

2. **To make the dough:** Stir together the flour, ground pecans, sweetener, salt, and butter. Mash the mixture evenly into a pie pan, pressing up the sides. It will be dry. Bake for 10 to 12 minutes, until golden brown. If the edges get too brown, cover with aluminum foil.

3. **To make the filling:** In a medium bowl, whisk the eggs and then add the pumpkin, sweetener, cream, pumpkin pie spice, pepper, and vanilla, mixing until incorporated. Pour into the pie pan, cover the outer edges of the crust with foil, and bake for 50 minutes. After baking, turn off the oven, prop open the oven door, and allow the pie to cool in the oven for about an hour.

4. **To make the sugar-free whipped cream:** In a medium bowl, combine the cream, sweetener, and vanilla, and beat on high for 1½ minutes, or until peaks form.

5. Refrigerate the pie and cream until time to serve. Slice pie into 8 slices, top each one with a dollop of cream, and serve.

COOKING TIP

An easy way to cover the edges of the crust when baking the pie is to make a shield out of aluminum foil. Tear a square piece of foil slightly larger than your pie pan. Fold the foil in half and then fold the long side in half again to make a square. Cut a large quarter circle off the corner and round the outside edges of the foil. Open it up and you'll either have a snowflake (oops, try again!) or an open hole in the center, in which case you can place it over the pie and tuck under the edges.

Per Serving: Calories: 391; Total Fat: 36g; Carbohydrates: 31.5g; Fiber: 6g; Net Carbs: 6.5g; Protein: 6g; Sugar Alcohols: 19g
Macros: Fat 83% Carbs 7% Protein 6%

Thanksgiving Leftovers Pizza

NUT-FREE

Prep time: 10 minutes | **Cook time:** 10 minutes | **Servings:** 4

Pre-keto, the best thing about Thanksgiving was the leftover turkey sandwiches on white bread with mayonnaise. It still sounds pretty good, but this Thanksgiving Leftovers Pizza is the bomb! I'll teach you how to make the crust from scratch, but we use Cutdacarb wraps, which you can order online for our family's make-your-own-pizza night. Feel free to improvise with your own leftovers, or add additional things like sausage or cheese. This recipe is for 4 servings, but you could double or triple the recipe depending on how many people you have to feed.

1½ cups grated mozzarella cheese

2 tablespoons cream cheese

⅓ cup coconut flour

2 tablespoons flaxseed meal

½ teaspoon garlic salt

2 large eggs, beaten

¼ cup (½ stick) melted butter

1 serving Green Bean Casserole (page 109)

1 serving Cheesy Mashed Cauliflower (page 112)

1 serving "Cornbread" Sausage Dressing (page 110)

6 ounces Roast Turkey, chopped (page 108)

2 servings Cranberry Sauce (page 113)

1. Preheat the oven to 425°F, and line a baking sheet with parchment paper.

2. In a microwave-safe bowl, melt the mozzarella and cream cheese in 20-second increments, until the mozzarella is melted and smooth. Stir together.

3. Add the coconut flour, flaxseed, garlic salt, and eggs, and work into a ball of dough. Wet your hands if it gets too sticky. Wrap in plastic wrap, and refrigerate for 30 minutes.

4. Spread out a sheet of parchment paper. Place the chilled dough on the parchment paper, and using a rolling pin or side of a drinking glass, roll into a round pizza shape or rectangle about ¼ inch thick. Using the parchment paper on the baking sheet, lay it on top of the dough and flip it over onto the baking sheet. Remove the top parchment paper.

5. Using the tines of a fork, poke holes throughout the dough. Brush on the melted butter, and bake for 7 to 10 minutes, until golden brown, rotating the pan halfway through.

6. Lay evenly across the crust, one of top of the other, the Green Bean Casserole, Cheesy Mashed Cauliflower, "Cornbread" Sausage Dressing, and Roast Turkey, and top with the Cranberry Sauce Place it back in the oven for 4 to 6 minutes, or until heated through. Use a pizza cutter to cut into 12 slices, and serve.

SWAP IT

Looking for other ideas for pizza ingredients? Some of our favorites are Alfredo sauce, cooked breakfast sausage, pepperoni slices, olives, jalapeños, shredded chicken, and all kinds of grated cheeses. Any of these would be perfect to add to this recipe or just to make an ordinary pizza. Always brown the flatbread first, then add the toppings, and pop back in the oven to heat.

Per Serving (3 slices): Calories: 514; Total Fat: 34g; Carbohydrates: 26g; Fiber: 9g; Net Carbs: 9g; Protein: 35g; Sugar Alcohols: 8g
Macros: Fat 60% Carbs 7% Protein 27%

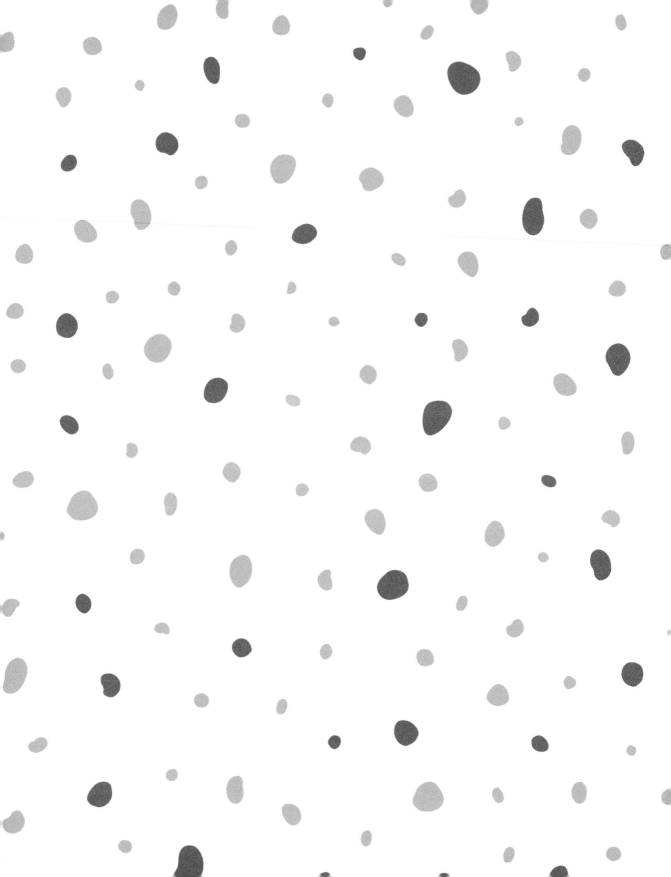

CHAPTER SIX

Winter Holidays

The winter holidays shine with a sparkle like no other, and the food of this season is, in a word, indulgent. We'll kick off December with a beautiful prime rib feast with all the trimmings fit for Christmas or Hanukkah that will leave you patting your belly in satisfaction. On its heels comes New Year's Eve, which we'll ring in with tapas, tidbits, and treats of all sorts, followed by a brunch the next day that will knock your socks off. We'll then prepare a Lunar New Year celebration full of foods that promise good fortune in the year ahead. The sweet ending to the winter season is a Valentine's dinner, featuring a rich and colorful array of keto-friendly foods that might just steal your heart.

A Very Happy Holiday Dinner

Crab Cakes and Sriracha Mayo (page 122)

Broccoli Cheese Soup (page 123)

Classic Prime Rib Au Jus (page 124)

Creamed Spinach (page 126)

Latkes with Sour Cream (page 127)

Pecan Pie Bars (page 128)

Baked Donut Bites with Jelly (page 129)

Latkes with Sour Cream, page 127

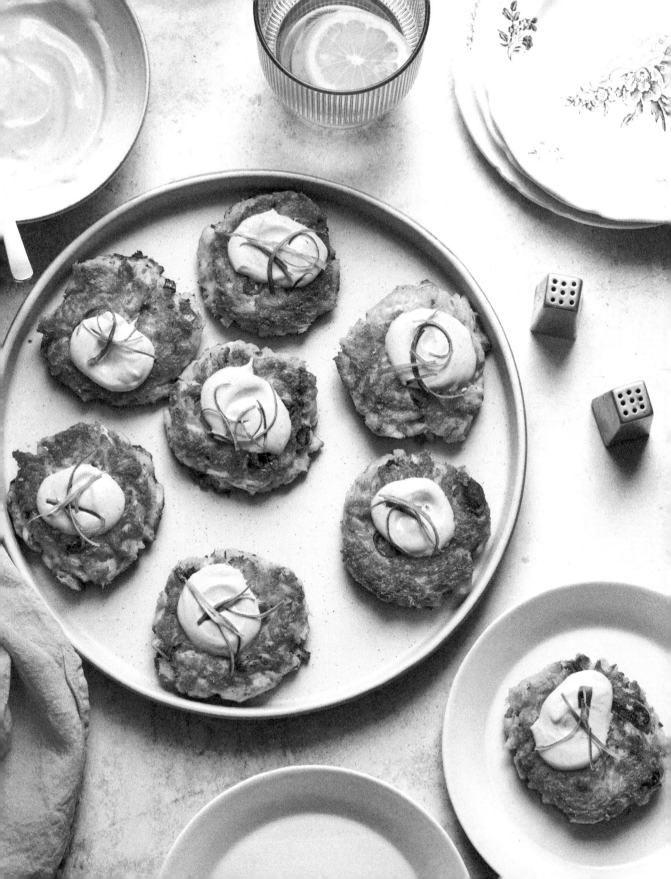

Crab Cakes and Sriracha Mayo

DAIRY-FREE

Prep time: 15 minutes | **Cook time:** 15 minutes | **Crab cakes:** 8

I love crab cakes. The crunchy outside and chunks of flavorful crab inside make a great savory appetizer or even a main course. They're super easy to make and so perfectly keto-friendly. They also make a very impressive statement for special occasions. I've paired them with one of our favorite sriracha-based sauces that you're sure to love.

FOR THE CRAB CAKES

½ cup peanut oil for frying

3 (6-ounce) cans premium lump crabmeat, drained

2 scallions, chopped

½ cup almond flour

1 large egg

3 tablespoons mayonnaise

1 tablespoon sriracha sauce

½ teaspoon freshly ground black pepper

½ teaspoon salt

¼ teaspoon garlic powder

FOR THE SRIRACHA MAYONNAISE

½ cup mayonnaise

1 tablespoon sriracha sauce

2 teaspoons pickle juice (dill or sweet and sour)

1/2 teaspoon minced onion

1. **To make the crab cakes:** In a medium skillet over medium heat, heat the peanut oil.

2. In a medium bowl, mix together the crabmeat, scallions, almond flour, egg, mayonnaise, sriracha, pepper, salt, and garlic powder. Divide the mixture into 8 portions, roll each into a ball, and pat into patties 2 to 3 inches in diameter.

3. Carefully place 4 of the patties in the oil. After 4 minutes, carefully flip each one and cook another 4 minutes. Turn the heat down just a bit, and place the remaining patties in the pan and repeat. Transfer to a plate lined with a paper towel to drain.

4. **To make the sriracha mayonnaise:** Stir together the mayonnaise, sriracha, pickle juice, and minced onion. Serve the crab cakes warm with sriracha mayonnaise.

SPICE IT UP

Kick the heat up a notch on either the sauce or the patties by adding some extra sriracha, red pepper flakes, or cayenne pepper.

Per Serving (1 crab cake with sauce): Calories: 251; Total Fat: 23g; Carbohydrates: 2g; Fiber: 1g; Net Carbs: 1g; Protein: 10g; Sugar Alcohols: 0g
Macros: Fat 82% Carbs 2% Protein 16%

Broccoli Cheese Soup

NUT-FREE

Prep time: 10 minutes | **Cook time:** 30 minutes | **Servings:** 6

I'm a soup lover from way back, and I believe there's none better than broccoli cheese. It's always so comforting on a cold night, and I swear it has magical benefits that can heal you when you're feeling ill. This recipe is super easy and cheesy good. I usually make a double batch 'cause it goes fast!

2 tablespoons butter

2 cloves garlic, minced

¼ small onion, chopped

½ teaspoon freshly ground black pepper

3 cups chicken broth or bone broth

1 cup heavy cream

1 (16-ounce) package frozen baby broccoli florets, thawed and chopped, or 3 cups raw broccoli

1 cup shredded carrots

1 teaspoon xanthan gum, optional

2½ cups shredded cheddar cheese

1. In a large pot over medium heat, melt the butter. Add the garlic, onion, and pepper, and sauté for 2 or 3 minutes, until translucent.

2. Add the broth, heavy cream, and broccoli, and bring to a boil. Reduce heat to a simmer, and cook for 10 to 15 minutes, until the broccoli is tender.

3. Add the shredded carrots and xanthan gum (if using), and then slowly add the cheese, ½ cup at a time, stirring constantly, until completely melted. Remove from heat and serve.

PAIR IT

This soup is super yummy paired with my Garlic Breadsticks (see page 165).

Per Serving (1½ cups): Calories: 416; Total Fat: 34g; Carbohydrates: 8g; Fiber: 2g; Net Carbs: 6g; Protein: 18g; Sugar Alcohols: 0g
Macros: Fat 74% Carbs 6% Protein 17%

Classic Prime Rib Au Jus

NUT-FREE

Prep time: 15 minutes, plus overnight to chill | **Cook time:** 2 hours 40 minutes | **Servings:** 8

When I was a kid, the holiday meats were such a big deal in our house. Always so much banter about how many pounds we needed to feed everyone, what method would be used to cook it, how long, what to season with, and so on. While turkey was the star for Thanksgiving, the prime cut of prime rib was the only choice for Christmas and required a field trip to the local butcher. To explain the hype, prime rib is the most desirable cut of beef with just the right amount of marbled fat—it literally melts in your mouth. Prime rib is definitely on the pricey side, so we want to be sure to cook it the best way possible. Don't worry, I've got you covered.

FOR THE MEAT

6-pound bone-in
  beef rib roast, tied,
  untrimmed
1 teaspoon salt
½ teaspoon freshly
  ground black pepper

**FOR THE
  HORSERADISH SAUCE**

1½ cups sour cream
⅓ cup prepared
  horseradish
5 teaspoons Dijon mustard
½ teaspoon salt
¼ teaspoon freshly ground
  black pepper
Chives, for garnish

FOR THE JUS

¼ cup red wine
2 tablespoons
  Worcestershire sauce
2 cups beef bone broth

1. **To make the meat:** The night before cooking, unpackage the meat, place it on a baking sheet lined with parchment paper, and place the sheet in the refrigerator, uncovered, to dry out overnight. (Note the weight before you discard the packaging.)

2. A half hour before you plan to cook your prime rib, remove it from the refrigerator. Season it with salt and pepper, and allow it to come to room temperature.

3. **To make the horseradish sauce:** In a small bowl, combine the sour cream, horseradish, Dijon mustard, salt, and pepper. Cover and place in the refrigerator.

4. Preheat the oven to 500°F. Place the prime rib on a rack in a roasting pan, fat-side up. To figure out how long to roast your meat, multiply the weight of your prime rib by 5, and this will be the roasting time. So for a 6-pound roast, you'll want to cook it for 30 minutes. Place the pan in the oven, and set the timer for the roasting time. When the timer goes off, turn off the oven, and don't open the oven door for at least 2 hours. After 2 hours, remove the meat from the oven to let it rest while you make the jus.

5. Take the horseradish sauce out of the refrigerator, and allow it to come to room temperature. Garnish with the chives.

6. **To make the jus:** Pour the drippings and browned bits from the pan into a medium saucepan over medium heat. Bring it to a simmer and whisk in the wine and Worcestershire sauce. Return to a simmer, and pour in the beef broth. Return to a simmer once again, stirring; then turn down the heat, and let it reduce, stirring occasionally, for a few minutes, until reduced by about half.

7. Remove from heat and pour it through a strainer into a bowl, using the back of a spoon to help mash it through. Carve the prime rib, and serve with jus and horseradish sauce.

PREP TIP

If you want to add more flavor to the meat, sliver some garlic, make tiny slits in the meat, and insert the garlic. It's so good!

Per Serving (6 ounces meat and jus and horseradish sauce): Calories: 386; Total Fat: 16g; Carbohydrates: 5g; Fiber: 0g; Net Carbs: 5g; Protein: 53g; Sugar Alcohols: 0g
Macros: Fat 37% Carbs 5% Protein 55%

Creamed Spinach

NUT-FREE, VEGETARIAN

Prep time: 10 minutes | **Cook time:** 15 minutes | **Servings:** 8

Growing up, we had creamed spinach and creamed corn at just about every holiday dinner. I haven't been able to keto-fy creamed corn, but creamed spinach was easy and tastes just as yummy now as ever before. I make a double batch for the holidays, but you can also cut the recipe in half, if you like. You can also make it more of a meal by adding some cubed grilled chicken.

½ cup (1 stick) butter, divided

¼ small red onion, chopped

3 cloves garlic, minced

1 cup heavy cream, plus more if needed

½ cup grated mozzarella cheese

1 ounce (2 tablespoons) cream cheese

½ teaspoon salt

¼ teaspoon freshly ground black pepper

¼ teaspoon xanthan gum

2 (10-ounce) packages baby spinach

¼ cup grated Parmesan cheese

1. In a medium pot over medium heat, melt ¼ cup of butter. Add the red onion, and sauté for 2 to 3 minutes; then add the garlic, and sauté for another 30 seconds. Pour in the heavy cream, mozzarella, cream cheese, salt, and pepper, and stir until mixed together. Using the back of a spoon, mash any cream cheese lumps. Reduce heat to a simmer, and add the xanthan gum, stirring while it thickens.

2. In another pan over medium heat, melt the remaining ¼ cup of butter. Add small batches of spinach to the pan to wilt, and cook until all the spinach is wilted.

3. Add the spinach to the cream sauce, and stir together. If it gets too thick, add a little more heavy cream. Sprinkle the Parmesan cheese on top, and serve.

SWAP IT
Instead of fresh spinach, you could use two packages of frozen spinach. Just be sure to thaw it and squeeze all the water out before adding it to the sauce.

Per Serving: Calories: 267; Total Fat: 26g; Carbohydrates: 5g; Fiber: 2g; Net Carbs: 3g; Protein: 5g; Sugar Alcohols: 0g
Macros: Fat 88% Carbs 4% Protein 7%

Latkes with Sour Cream

NUT-FREE, VEGETARIAN

Prep time: 15 minutes | **Cook time:** 45 minutes | **Servings:** 12

Growing up, whenever we had leftover mashed potatoes, my mom would make potato pancakes, or "latkes," the next day, and they were absolutely delicious. In this recipe, cauliflower makes for the perfect potato substitute!

1 (2-pound) head cauliflower, stems trimmed and florets coarsely chopped

2 tablespoons olive oil

½ teaspoon freshly ground black pepper

½ teaspoon garlic powder

½ teaspoon salt

½ cup grated mozzarella cheese

½ cup grated cheddar cheese

2 large eggs

3 tablespoons coconut flour

2 tablespoons mayonnaise

2 tablespoons olive oil, for frying

1 cup sour cream

2 scallions, chopped, for garnish

1. Preheat the oven to 450°F, and line a baking sheet with parchment paper.

2. Place the cauliflower in a gallon resealable bag, add the olive oil, seal, and massage and turn the bag to coat. Empty the cauliflower onto the baking sheet, and spread in a single layer. Season the cauliflower with the pepper, garlic powder, and salt.

3. Roast for 30 minutes. Remove from the oven, and when cool enough to handle, coarsely chop and place in a medium bowl. Add the mozzarella, cheddar, eggs, flour, and mayonnaise, and mix well.

4. In a medium nonstick skillet over medium heat, heat the olive oil. Using a large spoon, scoop the mixture, drop it in the pan, and pat down into a patty. Working in batches and being careful not to crowd the pan, cook for 2 to 3 minutes, or until golden brown on one side. Flip, and cook 2 more minutes on the other side. Remove from the skillet, and transfer to a paper towel–lined plate. Top warm latkes with a spoonful of sour cream and garnish with the scallions.

Per Serving (1 latke with sour cream): Calories: 156; Total Fat: 13g; Carbohydrates: 4.5g; Fiber: 1.5g; Net Carbs: 3g; Protein: 5g; Sugar Alcohols: 0g
Macros: Fat 75% Carbs 8% Protein 13%

Pecan Pie Bars

VEGETARIAN

Prep time: 15 minutes | **Cook time:** 40 minutes | **Servings:** 8

Pecan pie is one of my favorites, but until this book, I had made only one attempt at a keto-friendly version, which was an epic fail. This time, I asked to use a portion of my good friend Chef Taffy Elrod's Keto Pecan Pie recipe with a couple of tweaks of my own, and I think these bars are absolutely scrumptious!

2 cups coarsely chopped pecans

¾ cup coconut flour

¼ cup ground pecans

6 tablespoons melted butter

⅛ teaspoon salt

2 tablespoons granulated erythritol blend, plus ⅔ cup, divided

3 large eggs

⅓ cup sugar-free maple-flavored syrup

⅓ cup heavy cream

¼ cup (½ stick) melted butter

2 teaspoons vanilla extract

½ teaspoon salt

1. Preheat the oven to 350°F. Line a baking sheet and an 8-inch square baking dish with parchment paper.

2. Spread the coarsely chopped pecans evenly on the baking sheet. Bake for 7 to 10 minutes, shaking the tray halfway through. Remove from the oven, and allow to cool.

3. In a small bowl, combine the flour, ground pecans, melted butter, salt, and 2 tablespoons of sweetener. Mix into a dough, and press evenly into the bottom of the baking dish. Bake for 10 to 12 minutes, until golden brown.

4. Reduce the oven temperature to 325°F. In a medium bowl, mix together the remaining ⅔ cup of sweetener, eggs, syrup, heavy cream, butter, vanilla, salt, and chopped pecans. Pour the mixture over the crust in the baking dish.

5. Bake for 30 to 35 minutes, until golden brown on top. Remove from the oven, cool, slice into 18 bars, and serve.

Per Serving (1 bar): Calories: 197; Total Fat: 19g; Carbohydrates: 13.5g; Fiber: 3g; Net Carbs: 1.5g; Protein: 3g; Sugar Alcohols: 9g
Macros: Fat 87% Carbs 3% Protein 6%

Baked Donut Bites with Jelly

VEGETARIAN

Prep time: 5 minutes | **Cook time:** 10 minutes | **Servings:** 15

I love a cakey donut, and these baked donut bites, dusted with powdered sugar and served with strawberry jelly, are just delightful! These are my take on the traditional *sufganiyot*, or fried jelly donuts, eaten around Hanukkah, symbolizing the burning oil lamps in the ancient Holy Temple in Jerusalem. I chose to use strawberry jelly, but any flavor of sugar-free jam will work here.

Oil or nonstick cooking spray, for greasing

2 cups almond flour

3 tablespoons whey protein isolate, unflavored

½ cup confectioners' erythritol blend, plus 2 tablespoons for dusting

½ teaspoon baking powder

¼ teaspoon salt

4 large eggs

½ cup (1 stick) butter, room temperature or softened

¼ cup buttermilk

½ teaspoon vanilla extract

½ cup sugar-free strawberry jelly

1. Preheat the oven to 350°F, and lightly grease a mini muffin pan.
2. In a large bowl, sift together the almond flour, whey protein, ½ cup of confectioners' sweetener, baking powder, and salt. Add the eggs, butter, buttermilk, and vanilla, and mix well (it will be grainy).
3. Fill the muffin tins ⅔ full, and bake for 10 to 12 minutes, or until slightly golden brown. Remove from the oven, and allow to cool.
4. Spoon the jelly into a small microwave-safe bowl. Microwave for 10 seconds, and using a fork, mash it up so it has a more liquid consistency.
5. Transfer the donuts to a plate, and sift the remaining 2 tablespoons of sweetener over top. Serve with the warmed jelly on the side for dipping.

SPICE IT UP
To take your donut bites up a notch, you could also top them with blueberries, chopped pecans, sugar-free chocolate chips, or any other keto-friendly goodies you like.

Per Serving (2 donut bites with jelly): Calories: 185; Total Fat: 14g; Carbohydrates: 14.5g; Fiber: 1.5g; Net Carbs: 1.5g; Protein: 7g; Sugar Alcohols: 11.5g
Macros: Fat 68% Carbs 3% Protein 15%

New Year's Eve Cocktail Party

Baked Jam and Brie (page 132)
Antipasto Skewers (page 133)
Cheesy Baked Meatballs (page 134)
Sriracha Artichoke Bites (page 136)
Brown Sugar Bacon Smokies (page 138)
Sugar Cookie Balls (page 139)

Antipasto Skewers, page 133

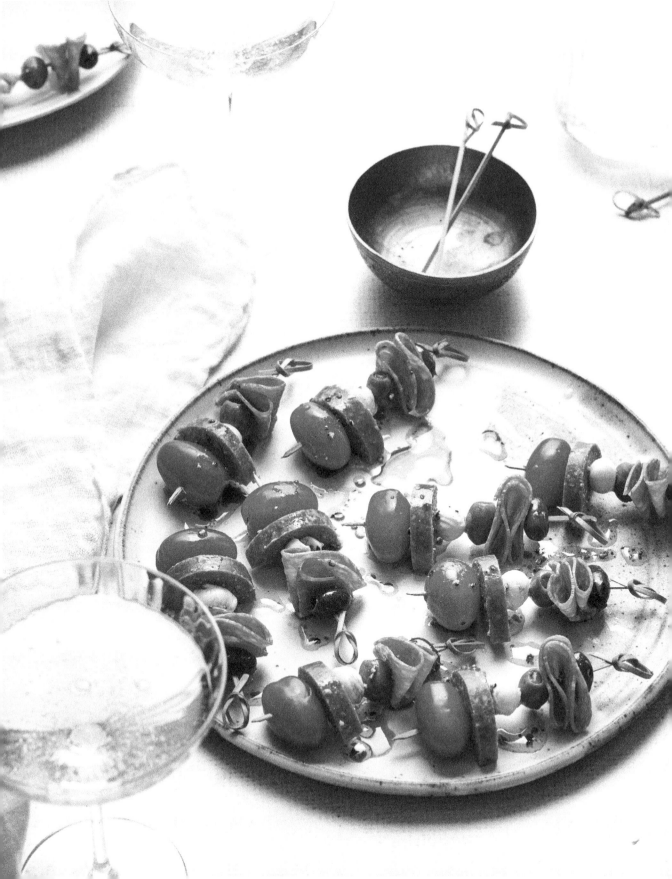

Baked Jam and Brie

VEGETARIAN

Prep time: 20 minutes | **Cook time:** 20 minutes | **Servings:** 12

Baked Jam and Brie has been my favorite appetizer, special occasion or not, for as long as I can remember. It's so festive and reminds me of the holidays. I used to make these with pie dough, which was full of carbs, so it was one of the first recipes I keto-fied. My favorite jam for this is Smucker's sugar-free blackberry, but you can use any sugar-free flavored jam you like. The "scoop," or holder, is formed using dough on the back of a mini muffin tray—you'll find the recipe for it on page 136 with the artichoke dip.

1 (6- to 8-ounce) package Brie

1 batch scoops (recipe on page 136)

½ (12.75-ounce) jar sugar-free blackberry jam

1. Preheat the oven to 300°F, and line a baking sheet with parchment paper.
2. Unwrap the Brie, cut off the white rind if desired, and cut into ½-inch cubes. Place a Brie cube in a scoop, place it on the tray, and repeat with remaining scoops and Brie cubes.
3. Bake for 3 to 5 minutes, or until the cubes have melted.
4. Place the jelly in a microwave-safe bowl, and microwave in 20-second increments until melted. Stir the jelly, and spoon some into each scoop on top of the Brie until they're full. Allow the jelly to cool, and set for 3 to 5 minutes before serving.

PREP TIP

You could also make this in one baking dish and serve it with crackers. You'll find the tip on how to make crackers on the page with the scoops. Lightly grease a small baking dish, place the cubed Brie in the dish, and melt in the oven or microwave. Then melt the jam and pour on top. Allow to cool and set, and serve with the crackers for dipping.

Per Serving (2 jam and Brie bites): Calories: 158; Total Fat: 12g; Carbohydrates: 6g; Fiber: 2.5g; Net Carbs: 3.5g; Protein: 8g; Sugar Alcohols: 0g
Macros: Fat 68% Carbs 9% Protein 20%

Antipasto Skewers

NUT-FREE

Prep time: 10 minutes | **Servings:** 12

Every time I serve antipasto skewers, I get so much praise for how pretty they are, and people ask me, "Where did you order them?" They're super easy to make and always present beautifully with their vibrant colors and textures. You can choose 5 to 7 of your favorite meats, cheeses, olives, fruits, and vegetables, taking into consideration size and color, and put them together in a flash. The hardest part is deciding in what order to place them on the skewer.

12 kalamata olives

12 slices thick-cut salami

12 pimento-stuffed
 green olives

12 marinated baby
 mozzarella balls

12 slices thick-cut
 summer sausage

12 grape tomatoes

1. On a 7-inch wooden or bamboo knotted skewer, thread the ingredients in this order: kalamata olive, salami (end to end), green olive, mozzarella ball, summer sausage (end to end), grape tomato. Repeat with the remaining skewers.

2. Plate and serve or store in an airtight container in the refrigerator until ready to serve.

PAIR IT

Drizzle these with some olive oil and balsamic vinegar, Italian dressing, pesto, or another sauce of your choice. You can also choose colors and foods that match the occasion or holiday. So much room for creativity!

Per Serving (1 skewer): Calories: 255; Total Fat: 22g; Carbohydrates: 2.5g; Fiber: 0.5g; Net Carbs: 2g; Protein: 11g; Sugar Alcohols: 0g
Macros: Fat 78% Carbs 3% Protein 17%

Cheesy Baked Meatballs

NUT-FREE

Prep time: 20 minutes | **Cook time:** 40 minutes | **Servings:** 12

I love serving fancy meatballs for a cocktail party, and these are so cheesy and delicious. They're perfect for New Year's Eve or any other party you have. They can be served up with a spoon or cute toothpicks or skewers, themed for whatever your occasion is. Make them in advance and simply heat them up so you can spend more time enjoying your party rather than working it! If you have leftovers, eat them over some baked spaghetti squash or zoodles, and voilà—dinner is served!

¼ cup olive oil, plus more for greasing

2 cloves garlic, minced

1 (10-ounce) can diced tomatoes with green chiles, like Ro-tel

1 (8-ounce) can tomato sauce

1 teaspoon salt, divided

¼ teaspoon freshly ground black pepper, divided

1½ pounds ground beef

½ cup crushed pork skins

¼ cup grated Parmesan cheese

1 large egg

½ teaspoon garlic powder

½ cup grated mozzarella cheese

½ cup grated Parmesan cheese

1. Preheat the oven to 375°F, and lightly grease a 9-by-13-inch baking dish.

2. In a medium pot over medium-low heat, heat the olive oil. Add the garlic, and sauté for 1 or 2 minutes. Reduce heat to low, and add the diced tomatoes, tomato sauce, ½ teaspoon salt, and ⅛ teaspoon pepper. Cook, stirring occasionally, while you make the meatballs.

3. In a large bowl, combine the ground beef, pork skins, Parmesan, egg, garlic powder, and remaining ½ teaspoon salt and ⅛ teaspoon pepper. Mix well, scoop, and roll into 24 balls about 1½ inches in diameter, and place side by side in the prepared baking dish.

4. Bake for 20 minutes, remove from the oven, cover with the sauce, and top with the grated mozzarella. Bake for another 20 minutes, covering lightly with aluminum foil if the cheese begins to get too brown. Garnish with the Parmesan, and serve.

PREP TIP

Double the recipe and make an extra baking dish of these to freeze for another day. After you cover the baked meatballs with sauce and cheese, let cool and then cover tightly with a layer of aluminum foil and freeze. Bake them from frozen at 375°F for about 30 to 40 minutes.

Per Serving (2 meatballs): Calories: 220; Total Fat: 15g; Carbohydrates: 3.5g; Fiber: 0.5g; Net Carbs: 3g; Protein: 16g; Sugar Alcohols: 0g
Macros: Fat 61% Carbs 5% Protein 29%

Sriracha Artichoke Bites

VEGETARIAN

Prep time: 15 minutes | **Cook time:** 35 minutes | **Servings:** 12

Artichoke dip is savory and fun, but add a little sriracha, and you've got a party! These artichoke bites are so easy and make a great presentation for a cocktail party. The "scoops" are made using the back side of a mini muffin pan as the mold; they can even be made in advance. They're a clever scoop for any dip or to fill with whatever you want—crab dip, chicken salad, taco meat and fixings are just a few of the many possibilities.

FOR THE SCOOPS

Oil or nonstick cooking spray, for greasing

1½ cups grated mozzarella cheese

2 ounces (4 tablespoons) cream cheese

½ cup almond flour

2 tablespoons flaxseed meal

¼ teaspoon salt

FOR THE ARTICHOKE DIP

Oil or nonstick cooking spray, for greasing

1 (14-ounce) can water-packed artichoke hearts, rinsed, drained, and chopped

½ cup sour cream

½ cup mayonnaise

1 tablespoon sriracha sauce

1 teaspoon garlic powder

¼ teaspoon salt

½ cup grated Parmesan cheese

2 scallions, chopped, for garnish

1. **To make the scoops:** Preheat the oven to 350°F, and grease the back sides of two mini muffin tins.

2. In a microwave-safe bowl, melt the mozzarella cheese and cream cheese in 20-second increments until the mozzarella is melted and smooth. Remove from the microwave, and mix in the almond flour, flaxseed, and salt, and work into a ball of dough (it will be greasy).

3. Spread a sheet of parchment paper on the counter. Split the dough in two, and place one on the parchment paper and one aside. Place another sheet of parchment paper over the top of the dough on the parchment paper, and with a rolling pin or side of a drinking glass, roll the dough out very thin, 1/16 to 1/8 inch thick. (The thinner you roll them, the crunchier they'll be.) Repeat this step with the remaining half of the dough.

4. Cut circles of dough using a 2¼-inch round cookie cutter or something similar. Set the muffin pans upside down, and place a circle of dough flat on top of each of the mounds. Repeat until all the tops are covered. If the dough circles touch each other, trim them smaller.

5. Bake for 10 to 15 minutes, turning the pans about halfway through, until completely golden brown. The dough will melt into a scoop. Remove from the oven, let cool 1 minute, and then gently pop them off and allow them to cool. Store in an airtight container until ready to fill.

6. **To make the artichoke dip:** Preheat the oven to 350°F, and grease a small baking dish.

7. In a medium bowl, stir together the artichoke hearts, sour cream, mayonnaise, sriracha, garlic powder, and salt.

8. Pour the mixture into the prepared baking dish, cover loosely with aluminum foil, and bake for 20 minutes.

9. Remove from the oven. When cool enough to handle, spoon the mixture into the scoops. Sprinkle with the Parmesan, garnish with the scallions, and serve.

PREP TIP

To make crackers instead, roll out the scoops dough very thin (¹⁄₁₆ to ⅛ inch thick), and then use a pizza cutter to cut vertical and then horizontal lines to make 1-inch square crackers. Place the crackers on a baking sheet lined with parchment paper, about ½ inch apart, and bake for 10 to 15 minutes, or until golden brown.

Per Serving (2 artichoke bites): Calories: 216; Total Fat: 18g; Carbohydrates: 6.5g; Fiber: 1.5g; Net Carbs: 5g; Protein: 7g; Sugar Alcohols: 0g
Macros: Fat 75% Carbs 9% Protein 13%

Brown Sugar Bacon Smokies

DAIRY-FREE, NUT-FREE

Prep time: 15 minutes | **Cook time:** 45 minutes | **Smokies:** 40

One of my favorite appetizers pre-keto was sweet and savory bacon-wrapped smokies rolled in brown sugar. They're a crowd-pleaser, and in my opinion, they should be served on every occasion, especially New Year's Eve. Luckily, these were easy to keto-fy! I just swapped the brown sugar for Swerve Brown, but you can use any brown sugar replacement that can be swapped 1:1. When shopping for cocktail smokies, or franks, choose the ones with the fewest carbs. My favorite brand is Hillshire Farms. This treat can be made ahead of time, frozen, and cooked right before your guests arrive—just add 5 minutes to the cook time.

¾ cup brown erythritol blend

1 pound bacon, cut into thirds

1 (14-ounce) package smoked cocktail franks

1. Preheat the oven to 400°F, and line a baking sheet with parchment paper. Pour the brown sweetener into a shallow bowl.

2. Wrap a piece of bacon around a smokie, roll in the sweetener, secure the bacon with a toothpick, and lay on the lined baking sheet. Repeat with the remaining bacon and smokies.

3. Bake for 30 to 35 minutes, until the bacon is crisp.

SPICE IT UP
Cut slivers of jalapeño and place on the smokies before you wrap them with bacon, or add a bit of cayenne pepper to your brown sweetener.

Per Serving (4 smokies): Calories: 187; Total Fat: 16g; Carbohydrates: 14g; Fiber: 0g; Net Carbs: 0g; Protein: 10g; Sugar Alcohols: 14g
Macros: Fat 77% Carbs 0% Protein 21%

Sugar Cookie Balls

NUT-FREE, VEGETARIAN

Prep time: 15 minutes, plus 1 hour to chill | **Cook time:** 10 minutes | **Servings:** 24

I have wonderful, vivid memories of making sugar cookies as a kid. They make the whole house smell like the holidays! This is a very easy version that I make in scoops rather than flattened, decorated cookies, but you can do that instead (see tip). This is a larger recipe for groups of people or to freeze so you can have sugar cookies anytime you please.

1 cup (2 sticks) butter

1 cup granulated erythritol blend, divided

5 large eggs

3 ounces (6 tablespoons) cream cheese, room temperature

1 teaspoon vanilla extract

1¾ cups coconut flour

2 teaspoons baking powder

⅛ teaspoon salt

1. In a large bowl, cream together the butter, ¾ cup of sweetener, eggs, cream cheese, and vanilla.

2. In a small bowl, sift together the flour, baking powder, and salt. Slowly add the flour mixture to the creamed mixture, and mix until incorporated. Cover with plastic wrap, and refrigerate for at least 1 hour so they don't spread while baking.

3. Preheat the oven to 350°F, and line a baking sheet with parchment paper. Using a cookie scoop, scoop the dough onto the baking sheet, 1 inch apart. Sprinkle the cookies with the remaining ¼ cup of sweetener.

4. Bake for 12 minutes, being sure not to overbake. Allow to cool on the baking sheet before removing. Store any leftover cookie dough in the refrigerator or freezer.

PREP TIP

If you'd like to make a traditional round, flat cookie, simply scoop the chilled dough, quickly roll it into a ball in the palm of your hand, and then flatten it to a ¼-inch-thick disc to bake.

Per Serving (2 cookie balls): Calories: 130; Total Fat: 11g; Carbohydrates: 13g; Fiber: 3.5g; Net Carbs: 1.5g; Protein: 3g; Sugar Alcohols: 8g
Macros: Fat 76% Carbs 5% Protein 9%

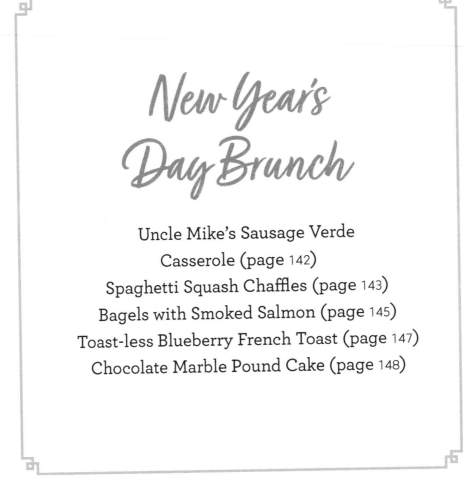

New Year's Day Brunch

Uncle Mike's Sausage Verde
Casserole (page 142)
Spaghetti Squash Chaffles (page 143)
Bagels with Smoked Salmon (page 145)
Toast-less Blueberry French Toast (page 147)
Chocolate Marble Pound Cake (page 148)

Toast-less Blueberry French Toast, page 147

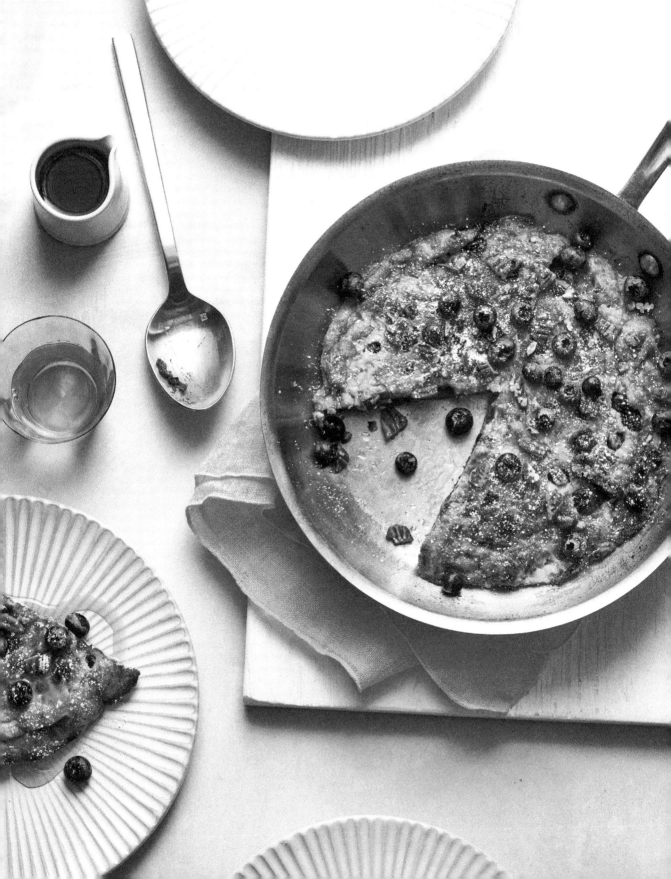

Uncle Mike's Sausage Verde Casserole

NUT-FREE

Prep time: 20 minutes | **Cook time:** 35 minutes | **Servings:** 10

New Year's Day brunch is a perfect time for Uncle Mike's (Lovies's brother) sausage verde casserole, but really, any day is good! Super easy and so full of flavor, it makes breakfast or brunch a deliciously memorable occasion. We love to make it all sausage, but you could also try it with half bacon, chorizo, or even hamburger. We also like to add a dollop of sour cream and hot sauce on top of each serving to make it look festive, but it's great all by itself. This big version ensures large servings and leftovers, so you could easily cut the recipe in half, but that would be silly!

Oil or nonstick cooking spray (optional)

2 pounds hot breakfast sausage, cooked and drained

18 large eggs

1 (11-ounce) jar green pepper sauce (see tip)

½ cup heavy cream

2 cups shredded cheddar cheese

¼ teaspoon salt

¼ teaspoon freshly ground black pepper

1. Preheat the oven to 350°F, and lightly grease a 9-by-13-inch baking dish or line with parchment paper.

2. In a medium bowl, mix together the cooked sausage, eggs, green sauce, heavy cream, cheese, salt, and pepper, and pour into the prepared baking dish.

3. Bake for 35 minutes, or until the center is cooked through. Serve warm.

PREP TIP
We like to use HEB That Green Sauce, but use whatever hot, medium, or mild brand of green sauce you like.

Per Serving: Calories: 566; Total Fat: 45g; Carbohydrates: 5g; Fiber: 1g; Net Carbs: 4g; Protein: 34g; Sugar Alcohols: 0g
Macros: Fat 72% Carbs 3% Protein 24%

Spaghetti Squash Chaffles

NUT-FREE, VEGETARIAN

Prep time: 10 minutes | **Cook time:** 1 hour 45 minutes | **Chaffles:** 6

Hash browns are something I dearly miss on keto. I played around with many foods and recipes hoping to find a hack to take their place but never quite hit the nail on the head—until these spaghetti squash chaffles! They've got a great flavor and that perfect crunchy texture that gives you the same savory feeling that hash browns do. They're wonderful as a "pusher" for eggs or just as a side. I like to make a breakfast sandwich with mine and add a fried egg and sausage. I used my Dash Mini Waffle Maker for these, but you could use a standard waffle maker as well.

1 small spaghetti squash (about 1 pound)
1 tablespoon olive oil
½ teaspoon salt, divided

Oil or nonstick cooking spray, for greasing
3 large eggs
½ cup grated mozzarella cheese

1 cup grated Parmesan cheese, divided
½ teaspoon garlic powder
½ teaspoon minced garlic

1. Preheat the oven to 425°F, and line a baking sheet with parchment paper. Cut the squash in half vertically, and scoop all the seeds and strings. Drizzle each half with the olive oil, and season with ¼ teaspoon of salt. Bake cut-side down for 30 minutes, flip, and cook another 10 minutes. Remove from the oven.

2. When the squash is cool enough to handle, use a fork to rake the squash strands into a small colander or cheesecloth. Mash or squeeze out as much of the excess water as you can; then place the squash in a medium bowl, and use a fork to pull apart the strands.

3. Grease and preheat a waffle maker.

CONTINUED

4. To the bowl with the spaghetti squash, add the eggs, mozzarella, ½ cup of Parmesan, the remaining salt, garlic powder, and minced garlic. Mix together well.

5. Drop two spoonfuls of the squash mixture onto the waffle maker, just enough to cover and fill the waffle plate. Sprinkle with a little Parmesan cheese, and shut the lid for 4 minutes. Open the lid, flip the chaffle over, sprinkle a little Parmesan across the top, close, and cook another 4 minutes. Repeat with the remaining squash mixture.

SPICE IT UP

These chaffles are delicious on their own, but you could also add some chopped green chiles or jalapeños to the mixture to take it up a notch or just add some sriracha on top when serving.

Per Serving (1 chaffle): Calories: 196; Total Fat: 15g; Carbohydrates: 6g; Fiber: 1g; Net Carbs: 5g; Protein: 9g; Sugar Alcohols: 0g
Macros: Fat 69% Carbs 10% Protein 18%

Bagels with Smoked Salmon

Prep time: 15 minutes, plus 30 minutes to rest | **Cook time:** 20 minutes | **Servings:** 8

Pre-keto, I was a bagel-and-cream-cheese junkie, especially with a little smoked salmon on top. There was just something so comforting about the thick, chewy bread and the cream cheese that made life a little better. There are many recipes out there for keto bagels, but I happen to think mine is one of the best—a bit of crunch on the outside and all chewy on the inside. Life is now complete with bagels back on the menu!

2½ cups grated
  mozzarella cheese
½ cup grated
  Parmesan cheese
2 ounces (4 tablespoons)
  cream cheese
1 cup almond flour
2 tablespoons
  coconut flour

2 teaspoons
  baking powder
1 teaspoon garlic powder
¼ teaspoon salt
2 large eggs, plus 1 egg for
  brushing on bagels
3 tablespoons Everything
  Bagel spice

4 ounces (½ brick)
  cream cheese
8 ounces smoked salmon,
  thinly sliced

1. Preheat the oven to 400°F, and line a baking sheet with parchment paper.

2. In a medium microwave-safe bowl, combine the mozzarella, Parmesan, and cream cheese. Heat in 30-second increments until the mozzarella is completely melted and smooth. Remove the cheese from the microwave, and stir to blend.

3. In a small bowl, stir together the almond flour, coconut flour, baking powder, garlic powder, and salt. Add half the flour mixture to the cheese mixture. Stir to blend. Add the eggs and remaining flour mixture, and mix together until incorporated. Let the dough rest for 30 minutes to make it easier to work with.

CONTINUED

4. Spread a sheet of parchment paper on the counter. With damp hands, make a ball out of the dough, and split it in half. Place half onto the parchment paper on the counter, and split the dough into 4 equal parts. Using your palms, roll each part into a 6- to 8-inch snake on the paper. Shape each dough snake into a circle on the baking sheet, pinching the ends to connect. Repeat with the other half of the dough until you have 8 bagels.

5. Whisk the remaining egg, and brush on top of each bagel. Sprinkle the bagel seasoning on each bagel.

6. Bake for 13 to 15 minutes, until golden brown, turning the tray halfway through the cook time.

7. Once the bagels are cooked, slice them horizontally. Spread 1 tablespoon of cream cheese on each bagel, top with 1 ounce of salmon, and serve.

SPICE IT UP
For extra flavor and fun, top with some drained capers and sliced red onion.

Per Serving (1 bagel with cream cheese and salmon): Calories: 338; Total Fat: 26g; Carbohydrates: 5.5g; Fiber: 2g; Net Carbs: 3.5g; Protein: 21g; Sugar Alcohols: 0g
Macros: Fat 69% Carbs 4% Protein 25%

Toast-less Blueberry French Toast

VEGETARIAN

Prep time: 5 minutes | **Cook time:** 10 minutes | **Servings:** 6

This is such a beautiful dish to serve for the holidays. I always place the pan on the table before I serve it because it looks so impressive. This flavorful dish tastes a lot like French toast, and it slices beautifully. I always make blueberry, but it would be equally wonderful with strawberries or any other berry.

1 tablespoon butter
6 large eggs
¼ cup almond flour
3 ounces (6 tablespoons) mascarpone cheese

7 tablespoons sugar-free maple-flavored syrup, divided
½ teaspoon cinnamon
½ teaspoon vanilla extract
½ cup blueberries, divided

¼ cup chopped pecans, divided
1 teaspoon confectioners' erythritol blend, for dusting

1. Preheat the oven to broil.

2. In a medium oven-safe skillet over medium heat, melt the butter.

3. In a medium bowl, whisk the eggs for 30 seconds, and then add the flour, mascarpone, 1 tablespoon of syrup, cinnamon, and vanilla. Mash and stir with a spoon until the bigger chunks of mascarpone are broken up. The mixture will be lumpy. Pour into the skillet, and cook, undisturbed, for 5 minutes. After the first 3 minutes, scatter half the blueberries and half the pecans over the egg mixture.

4. Transfer the skillet to the oven for 5 minutes. Remove from the oven, and scatter the remaining blueberries and pecans over top. Allow to sit for a few minutes, and then dust with the confectioners' sweetener. Cut into 6 wedges, and serve with a tablespoon of syrup on each slice.

PREP TIP
Make sure you're letting the dish sit for a few minutes before you dust it with the confectioners' sweetener so it doesn't just soak in and disappear.

Per Serving: Calories: 210; Total Fat: 17g; Carbohydrates: 7g; Fiber: 1.5g; Net Carbs: 2g; Protein: 9g; Sugar Alcohols: 3.5g
Macros: Fat 73% Carbs 4% Protein 17%

Chocolate Marble Pound Cake

NUT-FREE, VEGETARIAN

Prep time: 10 minutes, plus 1 hour to cool | **Cook time:** 30 minutes | **Servings:** 18

I love pound cake, any flavor, but chocolate marble is my weakness. I used to make it all the time (part of how I got in that mess), so when I started keto, there was a huge hole in my heart for its greatness. After playing around with recipes, I perfected one that would work for just about any flavor—and the chocolate marble flavor is our favorite. Baking it in a large rectangular dish feeds a bigger group and freezes well, but you could always cut the recipe in half and bake it in a smaller dish. To make it a little fancier, mix ½ cup of confectioners' erythritol with some water or sugar-free almond milk and drizzle it across the top!

Oil or nonstick cooking spray

¾ cup (1½ sticks) softened butter

1½ cups granulated erythritol blend, divided

10 large eggs

4 ounces (½ brick) cream cheese, room temperature

½ cup water

1 tablespoon vanilla extract

1 (13.66-ounce) can coconut cream

2 cups coconut flour

2 teaspoons baking powder

½ teaspoon salt

¾ cup unsweetened cocoa powder

1. Preheat the oven to 325°F. Lightly grease a 9-by-13-inch baking dish.

2. Using a stand or hand mixer, cream together the softened butter, 1 cup of sweetener, eggs, cream cheese, water, and vanilla for about 2 minutes. Add the coconut cream, and mix on low until incorporated.

3. In a small bowl, sift together the flour, baking powder, and salt, and mix. Add the flour mixture to the wet mixture, and mix on low for about 30 seconds, scraping down the sides with spatula, until incorporated.

4. Pour all but 2 or 3 cups of batter into the prepared pan. Into the remaining batter, add the remaining ½ cup of sweetener and cocoa powder, and stir together well. It should be thicker than the batter, but if it's too thick to mix, add a little more batter from the pan. Drop the chocolate mixture by equal spoonfuls across the batter in the pan, and use a knife to zigzag through the chocolate, back and forth, side to side, several times, to marble the batter.

5. Bake for 25 to 30 minutes, testing for doneness with a knife. If the knife comes out clean, it's done. If the top gets too brown toward the end, cover lightly with aluminum foil.

6. Remove from the oven and allow to completely cool before serving, at least 1 hour. It's actually best the following day.

COOKING TIP

You can also bake the full recipe in a loaf pan or Bundt pan or as cupcakes. If you're making cupcakes, shorten your cook time a bit. And if you're using a loaf pan, be sure not to whip the coconut cream with the butter and other ingredients, or the batter will grow in size and not fit into your loaf pan. I learned this by accident one time when I was in a hurry. (However, it did lead me to baking it in the larger baking dish, which has turned out to be our favorite!)

Per Serving: Calories: 239; Total Fat: 20g; Carbohydrates: 26g; Fiber: 6.5g; Net Carbs: 3.5g; Protein: 6g; Sugar Alcohols: 16g
Macros: Fat 75% Carbs 6% Protein 10%

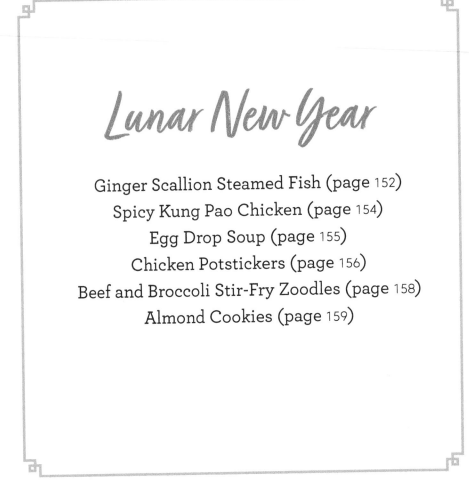

Lunar New Year

Ginger Scallion Steamed Fish (page 152)
Spicy Kung Pao Chicken (page 154)
Egg Drop Soup (page 155)
Chicken Potstickers (page 156)
Beef and Broccoli Stir-Fry Zoodles (page 158)
Almond Cookies (page 159)

Spicy Kung Pao Chicken, page 154

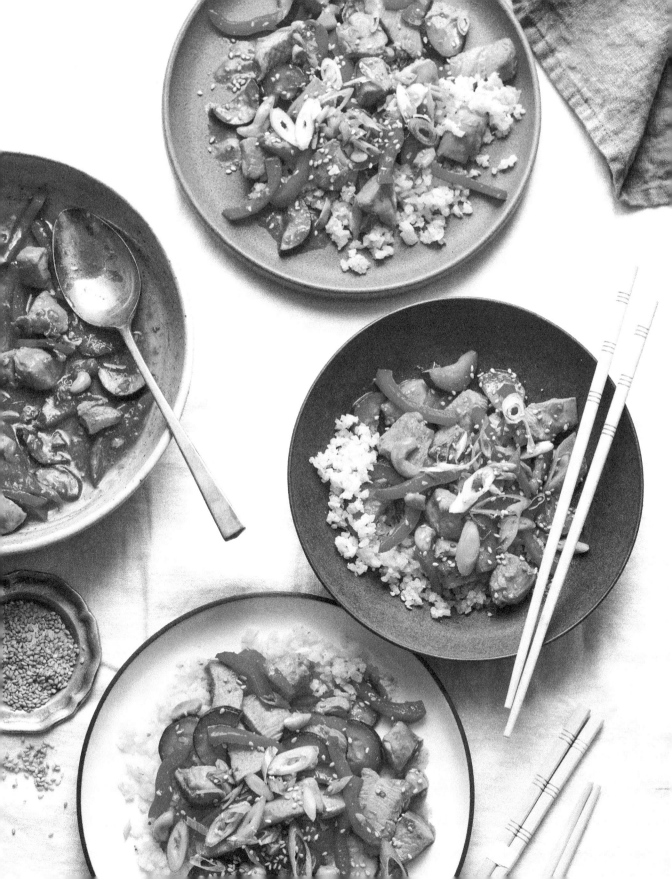

Ginger Scallion Steamed Fish

DAIRY-FREE, NUT-FREE

Prep time: 5 minutes | **Cook time:** 25 minutes | **Servings:** 4

I'd always seen whole fish in the market but never thought about cooking one or even how that would go. Steaming the whole fish represents unity in the Chinese culture, along with wealth and good fortune. I was impressed with how easily the recipe came together and just how delicious it turned out. You can use any kind of fish you like, but I chose tilapia. Steaming in a wok on the stove is more traditional, but steaming in the oven using a foil pouch is easier and works out wonderfully!

4 scallions, white part chopped, green part cut in 2- to 3-inch pieces and sliced lengthwise in half
2 garlic cloves, minced
1½ thumb-size pieces fresh ginger, thinly sliced

1 (4- to 5-pound) (or 2 smaller) head-on tilapia (or sea bass, catfish, flounder, or other white-fleshed fish), scaled, gutted, and patted dry

1 tablespoon soy sauce
2 teaspoons rice wine vinegar
2 teaspoons sesame oil

1. Preheat the oven to 400°F, and place parchment paper on a baking dish large enough to hold the fish, with a little extra room for the foil on the ends and sides. Lay a piece of aluminum foil, large enough to fold over the fish and seal, on top of the parchment paper.

2. Place one-third of the green and white scallions, garlic, and ginger across the bottom of the foil, and then place the fish on top. Open the fish cavity, and place another third of the scallions, garlic, and ginger inside. Close the fish, and top with the remaining garlic and ginger, reserving the remaining scallions for garnish.

3. In a small bowl, whisk together the soy sauce, vinegar, and sesame oil, and drizzle over the fish. Fold the foil over and roll the edges a couple of times to seal the foil pouch.

4. Bake for 25 minutes. Remove the foil, plate the fish, and sprinkle the remaining scallions on top.

COOKING TIP

You can always tell if fish is cooked through by whether it flakes. Poke the tines of a fork in the meatiest part of the fish and twist. If it resists flaking, put it back in the oven for a little longer.

Per Serving: Calories: 272; Total Fat: 6.5g; Carbohydrates: 2.5g; Fiber: 0.5g; Net Carbs: 2g; Protein: 51g; Sugar Alcohols: 0g
Macros: Fat 22% Carbs 3% Protein 75%

Spicy Kung Pao Chicken

DAIRY-FREE

Prep time: 20 minutes, plus 10 minutes to marinate | **Cook time:** 10 minutes | **Servings:** 6

I love kung pao chicken, and this recipe is better than any I've had from a restaurant. For even more flavor, let the chicken marinate in the sauce overnight. Traditionally, the cashews are left whole, but they're pretty carby, so to make them stretch, they've been chopped in half. If you're trying to cut your carbs, you can leave them out altogether.

- 1½ pounds boneless skinless chicken breast, cut into bite-size pieces
- 6 tablespoons soy sauce
- 4 teaspoons sesame oil
- 3 teaspoons sriracha sauce
- 2 teaspoons granulated erythritol blend
- 1 teaspoon fish sauce

- 1 teaspoon apple cider vinegar
- ½ teaspoon minced fresh ginger
- 1 medium red pepper, stem, seeds, and pith removed
- 1 medium zucchini, stem removed

- 2 tablespoons olive oil
- ½ teaspoon xanthan gum
- 2 ounces (20 to 25) cashews, halved
- 1 tablespoon sesame seeds, for garnish
- 2 scallions, chopped, for garnish

1. Place the raw chicken bites in a medium bowl. In a small bowl, whisk together the soy sauce, sesame oil, sriracha, sweetener, fish sauce, vinegar, and ginger. Pour 2 tablespoons of the soy sauce mixture over the chicken, stir, cover, and marinate for at least 10 minutes or up to overnight.

2. Chop the red pepper into bite-size pieces. Cut the zucchini into ½-inch slices and quarter each slice. Set aside.

3. In a large skillet or wok over medium heat, heat the olive oil. Place the chicken in the skillet, and cook, stirring occasionally, for 3 to 5 minutes, until cooked through. Add the red pepper and zucchini, and stir for another 2 or 3 minutes. Stir in the remainder of the sauce. Add the xanthan gum, and mix well with the sauce; then add the cashews. Stir for 2 to 3 minutes as the sauce thickens, and then remove from heat. Sprinkle with the sesame seeds and scallions, and serve.

Per Serving: Calories: 287; Total Fat: 15g; Carbohydrates: 9g; Fiber: 1.5g; Net Carbs: 6g; Protein: 29g; Sugar Alcohols: 1.5g
Macros: Fat 47% Carbs 8% Protein 40%

Egg Drop Soup

DAIRY-FREE, NUT-FREE

Prep time: 5 minutes | **Cook time:** 15 minutes | **Servings:** 6

Egg drop soup has got to be one of the easiest recipes out there. Most of the traditional recipes call for cornstarch to thicken them up, but I've found that unnecessary. It takes no time to prepare and always makes a beautiful presentation. To make it more of a meal, I'll add some shredded chicken or pork.

4 cups chicken broth or bone broth

4 cups vegetable broth

1 chicken bouillon cube

5 shiitake mushrooms, trimmed and thinly sliced

1 tablespoon soy sauce

1 tablespoon sesame oil

4 large eggs, beaten

2 scallions, thinly sliced, for garnish

1. In a medium pot over medium-high heat, combine the chicken broth, vegetable broth, bouillon cube, mushrooms, soy sauce, and sesame oil, and bring to a full boil.

2. Reduce heat to a simmer. Use one hand to hold a fork on the edge of the egg bowl, and as you gently stir the pot with the other hand, slowly pour the eggs through the tines of the fork into the hot water.

3. Pour into 6 bowls, top with the scallions, and serve.

COOKING TIP

This soup is best served immediately. If you want to make it in advance, you could have the broth, bouillon, mushrooms, soy sauce, and sesame oil all in the pot ready to boil, and then just add the eggs and scallions.

Per Serving (1½ cups): Calories: 112; Total Fat: 5.5g; Carbohydrates: 3.5g; Fiber: 1g; Net Carbs: 2.5g; Protein: 11g; Sugar Alcohols: 0g
Macros: Fat 44% Carbs 9% Protein 39%

Chicken Potstickers

DAIRY-FREE

Prep time: 15 minutes | **Cook time:** 50 minutes | **Potstickers:** 12

I don't know about y'all, but I can eat a whole plate of potstickers, no problem, and pre-keto, I did! Unfortunately, they're not even remotely keto-friendly, so here's my version that is delicious. I'm making them with chicken, but you could also go with a pork, fish, or even vegetable version if you'd like. Just watch your times so you don't over- or undercook your rolls.

FOR THE POTSTICKERS

1 large head cabbage
1 pound ground chicken
2 cloves garlic, minced
1 tablespoon soy sauce
1 teaspoon sesame oil
1 teaspoon sriracha sauce
2 tablespoons olive oil

FOR THE SAUCE

4 tablespoons soy sauce
2 tablespoons creamy peanut butter
1 teaspoon rice wine vinegar
1 teaspoon sesame oil
1 teaspoon sriracha sauce

1. **To make the potstickers:** In a large pot over medium heat, add enough water to fill the pot halfway. When the water begins boiling, place the head of cabbage in the water, core-side down, cover, and cook for 15 minutes.

2. Remove the cabbage, and when cool enough to handle, scoop or cut out the core. Carefully peel off the leaves. Choose 12 of the best leaves, and place on paper towels. Cut ½ inch off the cupped part (part of the leaf close to the core), and use the knife to shave across the rib/vein (without cutting the leaf in half) so it's easier to roll.

3. In a medium bowl, stir together the chicken, garlic, soy sauce, 1 teaspoon of sesame oil, and sriracha. Scoop a spoonful of the mixture into the cupped part of one of the leaves. Roll over once, fold in the edges, and continue rolling up. Repeat with the remaining mixture and leaves.

4. Add a couple inches of water to the large pot. Lightly grease a steamer (see tip), and set it in the pot of water. When the water is hot, place the rolls in the steamer, cover, and steam over medium-low heat for 25 minutes.

5. Place a plate lined with paper towels by the stove. In a nonstick pan over medium-high heat, heat the olive oil. When the oil is hot, add 2 or 3 rolls and panfry for 2 to 3 minutes, rolling them back and forth occasionally to get a good char on each side, and then transfer to the paper towel–lined plate. Repeat with the remaining rolls.

6. **To make the sauce:** In a small bowl, mix together the soy sauce, peanut butter, vinegar, 1 teaspoon of sesame oil, and sriracha. Serve the sauce with the rolls.

COOKING TIP

If you don't have a steamer, no problem. I've got a little campfire arts project that will do the trick. Make three balls out of aluminum foil, 3 to 4 inches tall (taller than the water level). Lightly grease a heatproof dish (a little smaller than your pot), and rest it on top of the foil balls. Place the rolls on the dish, cover, and steam.

Per Serving (2 potstickers with sauce): Calories: 229; Total Fat: 10g; Carbohydrates: 15g; Fiber: 5.5g; Net Carbs: 9.5g; Protein: 22g; Sugar Alcohols: 0g
Macros: Fat 39% Carbs 17% Protein 38%

Beef and Broccoli Stir-Fry Zoodles

DAIRY-FREE

Prep time: 10 minutes | **Cook time:** 15 minutes | **Servings:** 6

I love Chinese takeout, and one thing I really miss is stir-fry beef and broccoli over noodles. Well, crisis averted, because this recipe is so easy to make. If you're not familiar with spiraled zucchinis, your life is about to get a whole lot better. You can order an inexpensive spiralizer off the Internet, or you can use a vegetable peeler to make long and wide zoodles instead.

½ cup soy sauce

3 tablespoons rice wine vinegar

3 tablespoons sesame oil

2 tablespoons sriracha sauce

3 cloves garlic, minced

1 cup beef broth or bone broth

¼ teaspoon xanthan gum

2 tablespoons olive oil

1½ pounds skirt steak, thinly sliced across the grain, 3 inches long

1 head broccoli, cut into small florets, or 1 (12-ounce) bag frozen baby broccoli florets, thawed

2 medium zucchini, spiralized or cut into long strips with a peeler

1. In a medium pan over medium-low heat, whisk together the soy sauce, vinegar, sesame oil, sriracha, garlic, and broth. Cook, stirring occasionally, for 3 to 5 minutes. Add the xanthan gum; cook, stirring, for about 2 minutes, until it thickens, and remove from heat. Set aside.

2. In a large pan over medium heat, heat the olive oil. Add the steak and cook, stirring occasionally, until it begins to brown, about 5 minutes.

3. Add the soy sauce mixture, and stir with the steak. Add the broccoli and zoodles, and cook for an additional 3 to 5 minutes, or until the broccoli and zoodles are tender. Remove from heat, and serve.

Per Serving: Calories: 366; Total Fat: 26g; Carbohydrates: 7g; Fiber: 2g; Net Carbs: 5g; Protein: 27g; Sugar Alcohols: 0g
Macros: Fat 64% Carbs 5% Protein 30%

Almond Cookies

VEGETARIAN

Prep time: 5 minutes | **Cook time:** 15 minutes | **Servings:** 18

One of my favorite parts of Chinese buffets, pre-keto, was the almond cookies. It took many tries to keto-fy it, but I finally created what I consider a home run—these cookies have a wonderful, buttery almond flavor. During the Lunar New Year, Chinese almond cookies symbolize coins, so folks buy and eat them to bring good fortune.

2 cups almond flour

¾ cup confectioners' erythritol blend

½ teaspoon baking powder

¼ teaspoon salt

¼ teaspoon xanthan gum

2 tablespoons cold butter, cubed or grated

2 tablespoons buttermilk

2 tablespoons cream cheese, room temperature

½ teaspoon almond extract

18 almonds

1. Preheat the oven to 325°F, and line a baking sheet with parchment paper.

2. In a medium bowl, sift together the almond flour, confectioners' sweetener, baking powder, salt, and xanthan gum. Add the butter, buttermilk, cream cheese, and almond extract, and using your hands or a stand mixer on low, mix to incorporate.

3. Using a cookie scoop, scoop the dough, level the top with a knife, and roll into a ball in the palm of your hand. Place on the prepared baking sheet, and press down just a bit to make a cookie about 2 inches in diameter. Repeat with remaining dough. You don't need to leave much space between them; they don't spread. Press an almond into the center of each cookie for decoration.

4. Bake for 15 to 17 minutes, or until the edges are golden brown. They will seem undercooked, but don't overbake. Allow to cool completely before removing from the baking sheet. They will harden as they cool.

SWAP IT
You can also replace the almond with lemon or another flavor extract, leave off the almonds, and sprinkle with granulated erythritol on top prior to baking.

Per Serving (1 cookie): Calories: 87; Total Fat: 8g; Carbohydrates: 7.5g; Fiber: 1.5g; Net Carbs: 1g; Protein: 3g; Sugar Alcohols: 5g
Macros: Fat 83% Carbs 5% Protein 14%

Valentine's Day Dinner and Dessert

Strawberry Spinach Salad, page 164

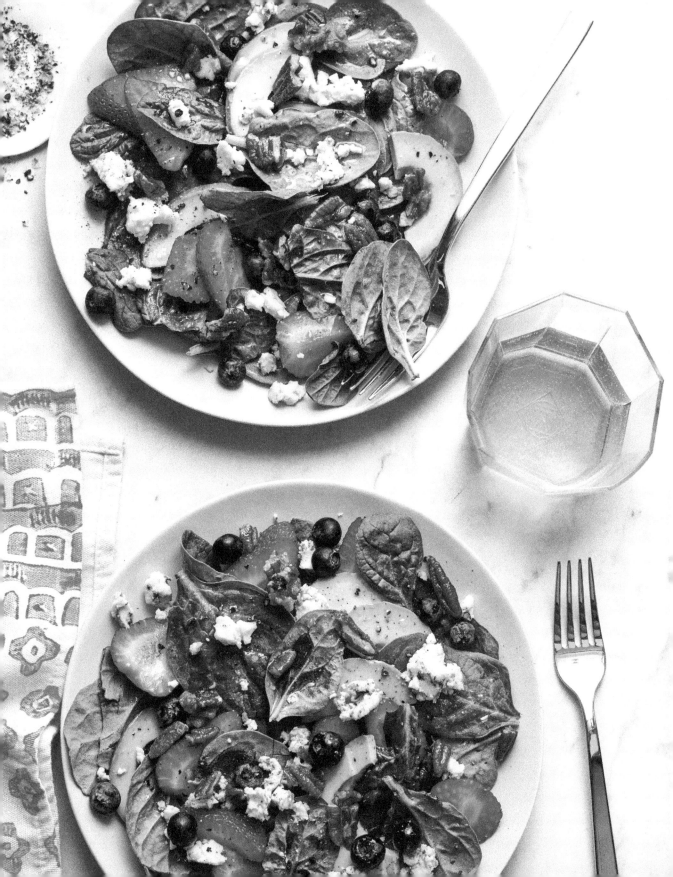

Salmon in Cream Sauce

NUT-FREE

Prep time: 10 minutes | **Cook time:** 10 minutes | **Servings:** 4

I love salmon prepared just about any way, but especially pan-seared. This method is the easiest way to really keep an eye on the fish and cook it to perfection. The cream sauce helps this beautiful dish really come alive!

1½ pounds fresh salmon, cut into 4 fillets, or 4 (5- to 6-ounce) fillets, about an inch thick, patted dry

1 tablespoon olive oil
¼ teaspoon salt
⅛ teaspoon freshly ground black pepper
⅓ cup sour cream

⅓ cup mayonnaise
½ teaspoon Dijon mustard
½ cup heavy cream

1. Heat a large nonstick skillet over medium-high heat.

2. Drizzle each fillet with olive oil, and season both sides with the salt and pepper.

3. Place each fillet, skin-side up, in the hot pan, and allow to sear, undisturbed, for about 4 minutes. Flip, and cook another 3 minutes, or until cooked through. Transfer the fillets to a serving plate.

4. Meanwhile, in a small bowl, whisk together the sour cream, mayonnaise, and Dijon mustard.

5. In a medium bowl with a hand mixer on high, beat the heavy cream until soft peaks form, about 1 minute, and fold into the sour cream mixture. Pour the sauce into the skillet and warm over low heat for 1 to 2 minutes. Serve the salmon topped with the cream sauce.

PAIR IT
I love to serve this over my Apricot Cauli-Rice Pilaf (page 177).

Per Serving (1 fillet): Calories: 530; Total Fat: 42g; Carbohydrates: 2g; Fiber: 0g; Net Carbs: 2g; Protein: 34g; Sugar Alcohols: 0g
Macros: Fat 71% Carbs 2% Protein 26%

Garlic Parmesan Asparagus

NUT-FREE, VEGETARIAN

Prep time: 5 minutes | **Cook time:** 10 minutes | **Servings:** 4

I love asparagus, especially roasted, and when you dress it up with garlic and Parmesan, it becomes special occasion–worthy. As fancy as it looks, it's super easy to throw together and pairs well with just about anything, especially Salmon in Cream Sauce (page 162)—the color and crunch of the asparagus perfectly complement the creamy salmon.

1 pound fresh asparagus, ends trimmed

2 tablespoons olive oil

1 teaspoon salt

½ teaspoon freshly ground black pepper

3 garlic cloves, minced

¼ cup grated Parmesan cheese

1. Preheat the oven to 425°F, and line a baking sheet with parchment paper.

2. Place the asparagus in a gallon resealable bag, and add the olive oil. Seal and massage the bag to coat the asparagus, and then empty onto the lined baking sheet in a single layer, with a bit of room between the spears. Sprinkle with the salt, pepper, and minced garlic.

3. Cook for 8 minutes. Remove the pan, sprinkle the Parmesan over the asparagus, and return to the oven for 2 more minutes. Serve warm.

PREP TIP

A fast and easy way to cut asparagus when cooking a larger bunch like this is to snap the end off one spear and then line up the rest and cut them all to the same length.

Per Serving: Calories: 96; Total Fat: 8g; Carbohydrates: 3.5g; Fiber: 1g; Net Carbs: 2.5g; Protein: 3g; Sugar Alcohols: 0g
Macros: Fat 75% Carbs 10% Protein 13%

Strawberry Spinach Salad

VEGETARIAN

Prep time: 15 minutes | **Cook time:** 5 minutes | **Servings:** 4

This salad makes such a beautiful presentation, especially for Valentine's Day, but it would also be great for any other occasion or even a weekday. With so many colors and textures, the berries, avocados, candied pecans, and blue cheese crumbles combine for the most delicious explosion of flavors.

FOR THE CANDIED PECANS

2 teaspoons butter

2 teaspoons brown erythritol blend

¼ cup chopped pecans

FOR THE DRESSING

3 tablespoons extra-light olive oil

3 tablespoons white wine vinegar

2 teaspoons granulated erythritol blend

1 teaspoon garlic powder

½ teaspoon minced onion

¼ teaspoon salt

⅛ teaspoon freshly ground black pepper

FOR THE SALAD

1 (10-ounce) package fresh baby spinach, torn into bite-size pieces

1 cup strawberries, cored and sliced

½ cup fresh blueberries

½ avocado, peeled, pitted, and cut into bite-size pieces

⅓ cup crumbled blue cheese

1. **To make the candied pecans:** Spread a piece of parchment paper on the counter by the stove. In a small pan over medium heat, melt the butter. Add the brown sweetener and pecans. Stir for 3 to 5 minutes, until the pecans are well coated and the sauce has thickened. Spread evenly on the parchment paper, and allow to cool and dry.

2. **To make the dressing:** In a small bowl, whisk together the olive oil, vinegar, sweetener, garlic powder, minced onion, salt, and pepper. Set aside.

3. **To make the salad:** In a large bowl, combine the spinach, strawberries, and blueberries. Add half the dressing and toss to coat. Top the salad with the avocado, candied pecans, and blue cheese. Serve with additional dressing.

Per Serving: Calories: 260; Total Fat: 23g; Carbohydrates: 14.5g; Fiber: 4.5g; Net Carbs: 6g; Protein: 5g; Sugar Alcohols: 4g
Macros: Fat 80% Carbs 9% Protein 8%

Garlic Breadsticks

VEGETARIAN

Prep time: 15 minutes, plus 30 minutes to rest | **Cook time:** 15 minutes | **Breadsticks:** 8

Best bread ever? I vote for garlic bread. It's great with soups, salads, or meals, or even cut in half for sandwiches. It's also one of the things I missed most when I started keto. After several attempts to get it just right, I think this recipe is sensational. The recipe makes eight 6- to 8-inch breadsticks, but you could make more smaller ones—even turn them into bread bites. I also like to roll them out longer and thinner and turn them into bread pretzels, like Auntie Anne's. If you make them smaller, watch the clock because they'll bake a little faster.

1 cup almond flour

2 tablespoons coconut flour

2 teaspoons baking powder

1 teaspoon garlic powder

¼ teaspoon salt

2½ cups grated mozzarella cheese

½ cup grated sharp cheddar cheese

2 ounces (4 tablespoons) cream cheese

2 large eggs

2 tablespoons garlic salt

1. Preheat the oven to 400°F, and line a baking sheet with parchment paper.

2. In a small bowl, stir together the almond flour, coconut flour, baking powder, garlic powder, and salt. Set aside.

3. In a medium microwave-safe bowl, combine the mozzarella, cheddar, and cream cheese. Heat in 30-second increments until the mixture is melted and smooth.

4. Remove the cheese from the microwave, and stir to blend. Add half the flour mixture, and mix. Add the eggs and remaining flour mixture, and mix together until incorporated. Let the dough rest for 30 minutes to make it easier to work with.

CONTINUED

5. Spread a piece of parchment paper on the counter. With damp hands, make a ball out of the dough, and split it in half. Place half the ball on the parchment paper on the counter, and split it into 4 equal parts. Using your palms, roll each part into a 6- to 8-inch breadstick. Place the 4 breadsticks on the baking sheet. Repeat with the remaining dough to make 8 breadsticks total.

6. Sprinkle the garlic salt over the breadsticks. Bake for 13 to 15 minutes, or until golden brown, turning halfway through. Remove from the oven, and serve.

PREP TIP
Don't forget to let the dough sit for 30 minutes—it's much easier to work with. Just keep your hands damp with water so the dough doesn't stick to them.

Per Serving (1 breadstick): Calories: 254; Total Fat: 20g; Carbohydrates: 4g; Fiber: 2g; Net Carbs: 2g; Protein: 14g; Sugar Alcohols: 0g
Macros: Fat 71% Carbs 3% Protein 22%

Chocolate Fudge

NUT-FREE, VEGETARIAN

Prep time: 10 minutes, plus 30 minutes to chill | **Cook time:** 5 minutes | **Pieces:** 12

Fudge doesn't need much of an introduction or story of "why I love it so much"—it's fudge; say no more! This is a super simple recipe, and I like to spoon it into silicone molds for the holidays to make cute desserts. A heart mold would be perfect for Valentine's!

½ cup (1 stick) butter
3 ounces
 unsweetened baker's
 chocolate, chopped

⅔ cup confectioners'
 erythritol blend
1 teaspoon vanilla extract
Pinch freshly ground
 black pepper

8 ounces (1 brick)
 cream cheese, room
 temperature

1. Line a small dish or pan with a piece of parchment paper large enough to hang over the sides.

2. In a medium saucepan over medium-low heat, melt the butter. Add the chocolate, and cook, stirring, until melted and incorporated. Remove from heat and stir in the confectioners' sweetener, vanilla, and pepper.

3. Add the cream cheese. With a hand mixer on low speed, cream together for 2 minutes. Spoon into the lined dish and refrigerate or freeze until firm, at least 30 minutes. Cut into 12 pieces. Leftovers can be stored in the freezer or refrigerator.

SPICE IT UP
Elevate the taste and visual appeal with a small amount of coarse sea salt flakes sprinkled on top. You can also stir in a swirl of peanut butter or add some nuts for a little extra flavor.

Per Serving (1 piece): Calories: 180; Total Fat: 18g; Carbohydrates: 10g; Fiber: 1.5g; Net Carbs: 1.5g; Protein: 2g; Sugar Alcohols: 7g
Macros: Fat 90% Carbs 3% Protein 4%

CHAPTER SEVEN

Anytime Celebrations

"Anytime" celebrations include all
the other occasions in your life deserving
of celebration-worthy food. For starters,
we'll plan a festive birthday dinner, complete
with a yummy frosted birthday cake! Then
we'll take the field with a game-day spread
that'll leave everyone doing the victory dance.
And finally, I've included a menu for bigger
groups. But don't expect leftovers—
these foods will go!

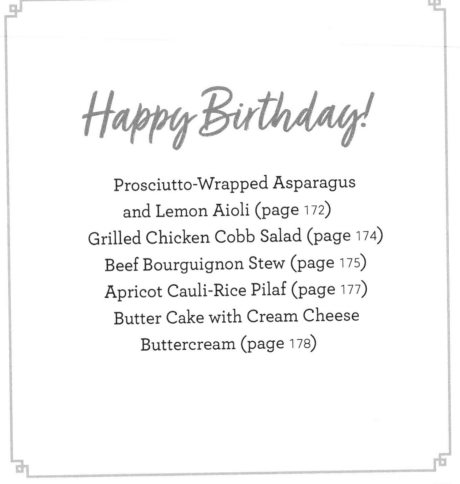

Happy Birthday!

Prosciutto-Wrapped Asparagus
and Lemon Aioli (page 172)

Grilled Chicken Cobb Salad (page 174)

Beef Bourguignon Stew (page 175)

Apricot Cauli-Rice Pilaf (page 177)

Butter Cake with Cream Cheese
Buttercream (page 178)

Butter Cake with Cream Cheese Buttercream, page 178

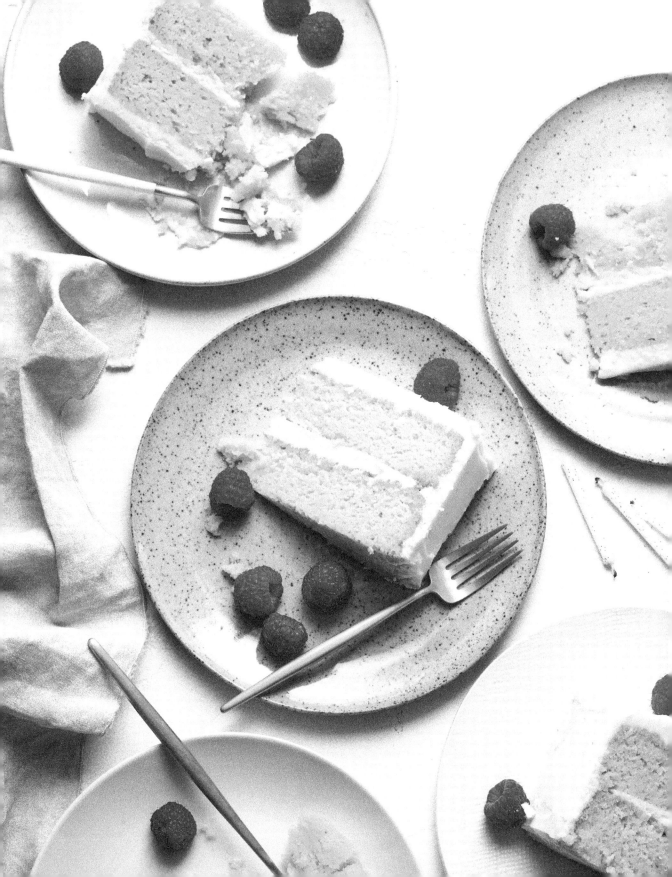

Prosciutto-Wrapped Asparagus and Lemon Aioli

DAIRY-FREE, NUT-FREE

Prep time: 10 minutes | **Cook time:** 5 minutes | **Servings:** 6

Asparagus wrapped in prosciutto is a brilliant combination. This recipe is my favorite all-time easy and fancy appetizer or side for any holiday or occasion. It takes minutes to prepare and is always a crowd-pleaser, with a delightful lemon aioli sauce.

½ cup mayonnaise

1 tablespoon fresh lemon juice, plus lemon slices, for garnish

1 teaspoon Dijon mustard

½ teaspoon garlic powder

¼ teaspoon salt

18 asparagus spears, trimmed to the same length

2 tablespoons olive oil

9 prosciutto slices, cut in half lengthwise

½ teaspoon salt

¼ teaspoon freshly ground black pepper

1. In a small bowl, make the aioli by mixing the mayonnaise, lemon juice, Dijon mustard, garlic powder, and salt. Set aside.

2. Preheat the oven to 425°F, and line a baking sheet with parchment paper.

3. Place the asparagus in a gallon resealable bag. Add the olive oil. Seal and massage the bag to coat each asparagus spear. Empty the asparagus onto the lined baking sheet.

4. Starting at the tip, wrap each asparagus spear with a piece of prosciutto, working at a downward angle to wrap, and place back on the baking sheet. Leave as much room between the spears as possible. Season with the salt and pepper.

5. Roast for 6 minutes, rotating the baking sheet halfway through and turning the asparagus.

6. Remove from the oven, and plate. Drizzle each serving with a table-spoon of aioli, or serve the aioli as a dip. Garnish each serving with a slice of lemon.

COOKING TIP
To roast a larger batch or if your baking sheet is too small to allow space between each asparagus spear, use two trays. This will help the prosciutto crisp up.

Per Serving (3 asparagus spears): Calories: 222; Total Fat: 21g; Carbohydrates: 3g; Fiber: 1g; Net Carbs: 2g; Protein: 7g; Sugar Alcohols: 0g
Macros: Fat 85% Carbs 4% Protein 13%

Grilled Chicken Cobb Salad

Prep time: 15 minutes | **Servings:** 6

I love a big salad, and this big Cobb salad with all the fixins is simply gorgeous. The colors and textures make this fancy salad a hit on any occasion. I like to make one salad in a pretty bowl and then toss and serve it at the table, but you could also prepare individual bowls—all up to you. The traditional Cobb salad is made with blue cheese crumbles, so if you want to go that route, add a few ounces of blue cheese crumbles to your salad and top with a dressing of your choice.

- 6 cups (2 large heads) romaine lettuce, chopped into bite-size pieces
- 8 ounces grilled chicken, chopped into bite-size pieces
- 8 cherry tomatoes, halved
- ½ small red onion, thinly sliced
- 1 avocado, peeled, pitted, and chopped into bite-size pieces
- 8 strips crispy cooked bacon, coarsely chopped
- 2 large eggs, hard-boiled, peeled, and coarsely chopped
- ½ medium cucumber, thinly sliced and cut in halves
- ¼ cup coarsely chopped pecans
- ½ cup dressing of choice

1. In a big serving bowl, evenly distribute the romaine across the bottom. Starting with the chicken, make a row across the bowl, and then follow with rows of tomato, red onion, avocado, bacon, eggs, and cucumber. Sprinkle the pecans evenly over the top of the salad.

2. Toss at the table, serve in bowls, and top with 2 tablespoons dressing, or more or less to taste.

SWAP IT
Put a seafood twist on this salad by replacing the chicken with shrimp.

Per Serving: Calories: 279; Total Fat: 20g; Carbohydrates: 8g; Fiber: 3.5g; Net Carbs: 4.5g; Protein: 18g; Sugar Alcohols: 0g
Macros: Fat 65% Carbs 6% Protein 26%

Beef Bourguignon Stew

NUT-FREE

Prep time: 20 minutes | **Cook time:** 2 hours | **Servings:** 6

There's no fancier stew than beef bourguignon, which is beef cooked in red wine. Julia Child made this stew famous, with the original recipe out of her book *Mastering the Art of French Cooking*. The world fell in love with her and her wonderful recipe, and I always feel so fancy when I prepare it. The stew traditionally includes pearl onions, but I left them out because they're a little carby, but if they work for your macros, feel free to add them in. You can also top each serving with a dollop of sour cream. That's my favorite way to eat this stew!

8 ounces bacon, cut into 1-inch pieces

3 pounds beef chuck, cut into 1-inch cubes

2 medium carrots, thinly sliced (¼-inch thick)

1 small white onion, chopped

3 cloves garlic, minced

2 teaspoons tomato paste

3 cups beef broth or bone broth

2 cups red wine

½ teaspoon xanthan gum

2 tablespoons butter

1 cup sliced white button mushrooms, cut in half

Chopped chives, for garnish

1. Preheat the oven to 375°F.

2. In a large Dutch oven or ovenproof pot over medium heat, cook the bacon until crispy. Transfer to paper towels to drain, reserving the grease in the pan.

3. Increase the heat to medium-high, and place a plate lined with paper towels next to the stove. Working in small batches, place the chuck cubes in the Dutch oven with the bacon grease, and sear on each side. Transfer to the plate with the paper towels.

CONTINUED

4. Reduce the heat to medium, add the carrots and onion to the pot, and cook, stirring, for 3 minutes. If the bottom of the pan is dark or crusty, add a table-spoon or two of water, and scrape up the bits.

5. Stir in the garlic and tomato paste, and then add the broth, wine, and xanthan gum. Stir for 2 minutes, and add the bacon and beef back to the pot. Cover and place in the oven for 1½ hours, stirring every 30 minutes.

6. About 15 minutes before the stew is done, in a small skillet over medium heat, melt the butter. Add the mushrooms, sauté for about 5 minutes, or until soft, and then set aside. Serve the stew topped with the mushrooms and chives.

COOKING TIP
If you want the bacon to stay crispier, wait to top the stew with it (along with the mushrooms) at the end.

Per Serving (1½ cups): Calories: 582; Total Fat: 30g; Carbohydrates: 8.5g; Fiber: 1g; Net Carbs: 7.5g; Protein: 56g; Sugar Alcohols: 0g
Macros: Fat 46% Carbs 5% Protein 38%

Apricot Cauli-Rice Pilaf

VEGETARIAN

Prep time: 5 minutes | **Cook time:** 45 minutes | **Servings:** 6

Apricot rice pilaf was first introduced to me by my dad's wife, Bev (Grandma Bev to the kiddos). Her version contained rice, pieces of apricot, and pine nuts, and it was not too sweet—just a delightful dish that made a fantastic side. To replicate this dish and make it keto, I made a few adjustments and am thrilled with how it turned out. If you'd like to add a little heat, you could sprinkle in just a bit of cayenne pepper.

1 large cauliflower head
2 tablespoons olive oil
½ teaspoon salt

¼ teaspoon freshly ground black pepper
2 tablespoons butter

1 tablespoon sugar-free apricot preserves
¼ cup pine nuts

1. Preheat the oven to 425°F, and line a baking sheet with parchment paper.

2. Pull off the cauliflower leaves and cut off the stems. Coarsely chop the florets and place in a gallon resealable bag with the olive oil. Seal, and massage and turn the bag until the cauliflower is coated.

3. Empty the cauliflower onto the lined baking sheet, season with the salt and pepper, and bake for 35 minutes, turning the baking sheet halfway through. Remove from the oven, and when cool enough to handle, place the cauliflower on a cutting board and roughly chop into rice-like pieces.

4. In a large skillet over medium heat, melt the butter. Add the apricot preserves, and stir for a minute until incorporated. Add the nuts, and stir for another 2 to 3 minutes, until they're well coated. Add the cauliflower, and stir constantly for 3 more minutes. Remove from heat, and serve.

SWAP IT
Try chopped pecans instead of pine nuts—they're a little less carby.

Per Serving: Calories: 144; Total Fat: 12g; Carbohydrates: 8.5g; Fiber: 3.5g; Net Carbs: 5g; Protein: 3g; Sugar Alcohols: 0g
Macros: Fat 75% Carbs 14% Protein 8%

Butter Cake with Cream Cheese Buttercream

VEGETARIAN

Prep time: 20 minutes, plus 1 hour to chill | **Cook time:** 35 minutes | **Slices:** 16

When it comes to birthday cake, let's just say I have some experience. With six years in the specialty cake business, I've made a few! This recipe is a simple butter cake that can be made into whatever flavor you like by adding a little lemon, orange, or whatever extract you choose. When this cake comes out of the oven, it will seem spongy on top and greasy, but just give it time to cool, and the magic will happen. For a little extra flair, you can decorate the top of the cake with strawberries, chopped nuts, or even some sugar-free chocolate shavings!

FOR THE CAKE
1¼ cups (2½ sticks) butter, room temperature or softened, plus more for greasing
6 large eggs
¾ cup buttermilk
⅔ cup water
1 teaspoon vanilla extract
4 cups almond flour

1 cup confectioners' erythritol blend
3 teaspoons baking powder

FOR THE ICING
16 ounces (2 bricks) cream cheese, room temperature

1 cup butter, room temperature
1⅓ cups confectioners' erythritol blend
2 tablespoons water
½ teaspoon vanilla extract

1. **To make the cake:** Preheat the oven to 325°F, and lightly grease the sides of two 8-inch round cake pans with straight edges. Cut out two circles of parchment paper the size of the cake pan, and place one in the bottom of each pan.

2. In a large bowl, use a stand or hand mixer to cream the butter until fluffy. Add the eggs, buttermilk, water, and vanilla, and mix.

3. In a medium bowl, sift together the almond flour, sweetener, and baking powder. Slowly add the dry mixture to the wet mixture, and mix for 2 minutes on slow to medium speed.

4. Pour the batter into the prepared pans and bake for 35 to 40 minutes, rotating the pans halfway through. When the top gets brown, test for doneness with a knife. The cake will seem jiggly, but if the knife comes out clean, it's done.

5. Allow the cakes to cool completely in the pans. Once cool, run a knife along the edge of each pan to help the cake come out of the pan cleanly. Wrap the cooled cakes in plastic wrap, and place in the refrigerator for 30 minutes or longer.

6. **To make the icing:** With a stand or hand mixer, combine the cream cheese and butter, and beat until fluffy. Add the sweetener, water, and vanilla, and beat on high for 1 minute.

7. Transfer the cake to a flat plate or cake board. Using an icing spatula or knife, spread a ¼-inch layer of icing evenly across the top of the cake, being sure not to get crumbs in your icing (see tip). Evenly rest the top layer of cake over the iced cake. Spread a very thin layer of icing over the top and sides. Refrigerate for 30 minutes, and then spread another coating of icing over the cake. Slice into 16 slices and serve.

PREP TIP

As you spread the first coat of icing (called the "dirty ice"), scrape the knife off in between each spread to remove any crumbs. Don't place a crumby knife back in the icing, or you'll have crumbs all over your icing! The second coat of icing should go on much cleaner, since it's coating icing, not cake!

Per Serving (1 slice): Calories: 502; Total Fat: 50g; Carbohydrates: 24g; Fiber: 3g; Net Carbs: 3.5g; Protein: 10g; Sugar Alcohols: 17.5g
Macros: Fat 90% Carbs 3% Protein 8%

Game Day!

Pigs in a Blanket, page 185

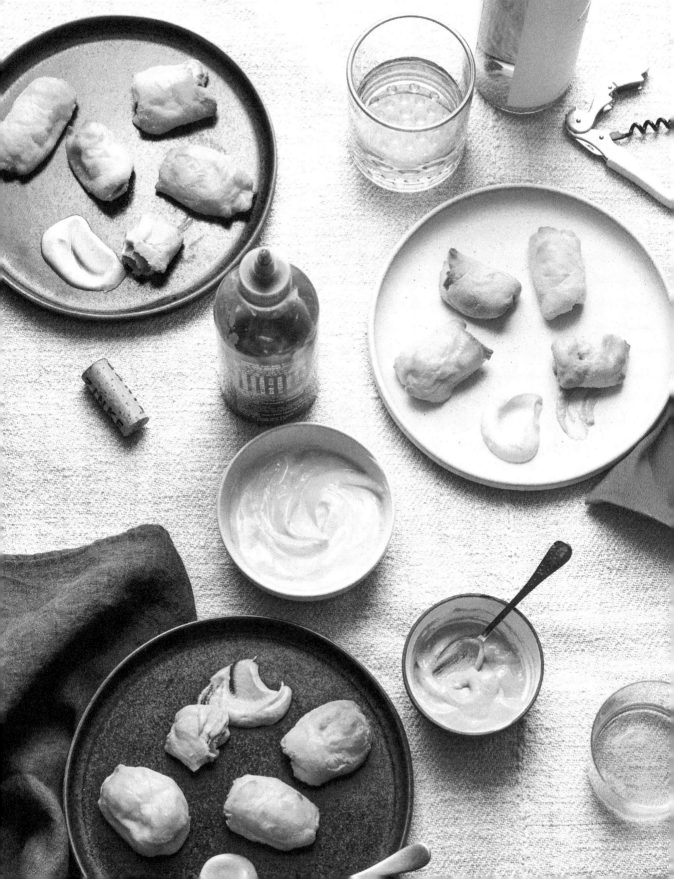

Spicy Jalapeño Chips and Ranch

NUT-FREE, VEGETARIAN

Prep time: 5 minutes | **Cook time:** 20 minutes | **Servings:** 8

I'm a "chip and dipper" from way back, especially when you add a little heat and some ranch. This recipe can easily be made in advance of the big game. You might even get one of the variety party packages of precut cheese and make an assortment. So many options!

5 medium jalapeños, very thinly sliced, with or without seeds depending on taste

1 tablespoon olive oil

½ teaspoon garlic powder

½ teaspoon minced onion

1 (7-ounce) package Havarti cheese slices

½ packet ranch dressing mix

½ cup sour cream

½ cup mayonnaise

1 tablespoon jalapeño juice, from a jar, or more or less

1. Preheat the oven to 450°F, line a baking sheet with parchment paper, and place a paper towel on a plate.

2. Place the sliced jalapeños in a resealable bag with the olive oil. Seal, and massage and turn the bag to coat the slices. Empty out on the lined baking sheet, spreading them flat, and then season with the garlic powder and minced onion.

3. Roast for 10 to 15 minutes, until crisp. Remove from the oven, and transfer onto the paper towel. Place a new parchment paper on the baking sheet, and reduce the oven temperature to 400°F.

4. Cut the cheese slices into quarters, and place on the lined baking sheet with a little space between them. Place a jalapeño slice in the middle of each piece of cheese.

5. Bake for 5 to 7 minutes, or until the edges are brown. Watch them because they'll burn quickly. Remove from the oven, allow to cool for a few minutes, and then transfer to a plate or bowl.

6. While the cheese is roasting or even the day or night before, mix the dip. In a small bowl, stir together the ranch dressing mix, sour cream, mayonnaise, and jalapeño juice. Serve with the jalapeño cheese chips.

Per Serving (5 chips with dip): Calories: 251; Total Fat: 23g; Carbohydrates: 3.5g; Fiber: 0g; Net Carbs: 3.5g; Protein: 6g; Sugar Alcohols: 0g
Macros: Fat 82% Carbs 6% Protein 10%

Pizza Pull-Apart Bread

Prep time: 15 minutes, plus 30 minutes to chill | **Cook time:** 30 minutes | **Servings:** 8

I can remember when pull-apart bread came to be, and folks were making pull-apart bread everything! Just pull off a piece, and off you go. This pizza pull-apart version is so easy and can be made in so many versions. I chose sausage and pepperoni, but you could add chicken, olives, mushrooms, bacon—anything you like. I serve it with Bertolli Garlic Alfredo Sauce (naturally low in carbs), but you could serve it with a low-carb marinara or even ranch dressing. It's all good!

- Oil or nonstick cooking spray, for greasing
- 2½ cups grated mozzarella cheese
- 2 ounces (4 tablespoons) cream cheese
- 1¼ cups almond flour
- 2 tablespoons flaxseed meal
- 2 tablespoons coconut flour
- 2 large eggs
- 2 tablespoons whey protein isolate, unflavored
- 2 tablespoons finely grated Parmesan cheese
- 1 tablespoon baking powder
- ¼ teaspoon garlic salt
- 1 pound pork breakfast sausage, cooked and drained
- 30 pepperoni slices

1. Preheat the oven to 350°F, and grease a Bundt pan with butter or non-stick spray.

2. In a microwave-safe dish, combine the mozzarella and cream cheese, and heat in 20-second increments until the mozzarella is melted and smooth. Remove and mix together.

3. Add the almond flour, flaxseed, coconut flour, and eggs. Using your hands, mix it together and then into a ball, and place the ball in the refrigerator for at least 30 minutes or longer.

4. In a small bowl, mix together the whey protein, Parmesan, baking powder, and garlic salt. Set aside.

CONTINUED

5. Spread a piece of parchment paper on the counter. Remove the dough from the refrigerator, and divide in half. Over the parchment, continue to halve each piece of dough until you have 32 equal portions, and then roll each of those into a ball. Roll each ball in the baking powder mixture, and set aside.

6. Evenly place a quarter of the sausage and pepperoni in the bottom of the Bundt pan, and then add 8 of the balls. Sprinkle in half the cheese, and then repeat, evenly adding more sausage, pepperoni, balls, and cheese, until it's all in the pan.

7. Bake for 30 minutes. Remove from the oven, run a knife around the inside of the pan to make sure the bread will pull apart from the sides, and then place a plate on the top and flip it over. If you think the bottom looks prettier, put another plate on the bread and flip it over again so the bottom side is up.

COOKING TIP
The first time I made this, I cooked the pepperoni first for 5 minutes and blotted off the grease and then added it to the pull-apart bread. It came out a little dry. The next time I left it uncooked, and the grease added a lot of flavor and moistness. So, whatever meat you use, consider not draining it all the way.

Per Serving: Calories: 456; Total Fat: 36g; Carbohydrates: 6g; Fiber: 3g; Net Carbs: 3g; Protein: 26g; Sugar Alcohols: 0g
Macros: Fat 71% Carbs 3% Protein 23%

Pigs in a Blanket

NUT-FREE

Prep time: 10 minutes, plus 15 minutes to sit | **Cook time:** 25 minutes | **Servings:** 9

I can remember going to the donut shop every Saturday morning as a kid and then with my son when he was a kid. The smell of fresh donuts and pigs in a blanket (also called sausage kolaches here in Texas) was the best—yes, our donut shop sold both! This was such an easy recipe to keto-fy, and now we make these all the time on the weekends.

2 cups grated mozzarella cheese

2½ ounces (5 tablespoons) cream cheese

½ cup coconut flour

1 large egg

½ teaspoon garlic salt

6 smoked sausages, cut into thirds (check the carb count)

1. Preheat the oven to 350°F, and line a baking sheet with parchment paper.

2. In a large microwave-safe bowl, combine the mozzarella and cream cheese, and melt in 20-second increments until the mozzarella is melted and smooth. Remove from the microwave, and mix together.

3. Add the flour, egg, and garlic salt, mixing well with your hands. Using your hands, form into a ball of dough. Allow to sit for about 15 minutes.

4. Divide the dough in half and then half again and again, until you have 18 sections. With damp hands, roll a dough section into a ball, place the ball in the palm of your hand, and flatten it out. Place a sausage on the dough, and wrap the dough around the sausage completely. Place on the lined baking sheet, and repeat with the remaining dough and sausage.

5. Bake for 20 to 25 minutes, or until golden brown, rotating the pan halfway through. Serve warm.

PREP TIP
You may want to wear disposable gloves to mix the dough so it won't stick to your hands.

Per Serving (2 pigs): Calories: 187; Total Fat: 14g; Carbohydrates: 5g; Fiber: 2.5g; Net Carbs: 2.5g; Protein: 10g; Sugar Alcohols: 0g
Macros: Fat 67% Carbs 5% Protein 21%

Sriracha Wings

DAIRY-FREE, NUT-FREE

Prep time: 10 minutes | **Cook time:** 1 hour | **Servings:** 5

Wingstop is one of my guilty pleasures and one of the reasons that I was able to stick with keto in the beginning. Anytime I got weak, I'd head to Wingstop and order a mess of wings, and it would detour any ideas of eating off-plan. Thank goodness wings are keto-friendly and just as easy to make at home. I love many different versions, but sriracha is one of my favorites. If you like heat, make these even hotter by adding some red pepper flakes!

- 1 (2½-pound) package chicken wings (20 to 22 wings), patted dry
- 1 tablespoon garlic powder
- 1 tablespoon baking powder
- ½ teaspoon salt
- ¼ teaspoon freshly ground black pepper
- ½ cup sriracha sauce
- 1 teaspoon sesame oil
- 1 teaspoon soy sauce
- 1 teaspoon brown erythritol blend
- 2 tablespoons sesame seeds, for garnish

1. Preheat the oven to 425°F, and line a baking sheet with parchment paper. Spread the chicken wings on the lined baking sheet.

2. In a small bowl, stir together the garlic powder, baking powder, salt, and pepper. Sprinkle half the mixture evenly on top of the chicken wings, flip them over, and sprinkle with the other half of the mixture.

3. Bake for 25 minutes, flip the wings over, and cook for 25 minutes more.

4. In a medium bowl, whisk together the sriracha, sesame oil, soy sauce, and brown sweetener.

5. Dip the wings in the mixture to coat evenly, and place back on the baking sheet. Bake for another 10 minutes and remove from the oven. Garnish with sesame seeds and serve.

PAIR IT
These wings are great served with your favorite ranch or blue cheese dressing. Add an ice-cold low-carb beer, and now you're talking!

Per Serving (4 wings): Calories: 299; Total Fat: 21g; Carbohydrates: 6.5g; Fiber: 0.5g; Net Carbs: 5g; Protein: 26g; Sugar Alcohols: 1g
Macros: Fat 63% Carbs 7% Protein 35%

Slow Cooker White Chicken Chili

NUT-FREE

Prep time: 5 minutes | **Cook time:** 3 hours 30 minutes | **Servings:** 6

Whether it's cold or hot outside, everyone loves chili at my house. When I was growing up, my mother made it all the time, and when I started keto, I wanted to be sure to have a version available that we all could enjoy—thankfully I came up with a white version that is so savory and good! We usually serve it up with a big dollop of sour cream on top. You could also add some sriracha to spice it up a bit.

- 2 pounds boneless, skinless chicken breasts
- 1 (4-ounce) can chopped green chiles
- ½ small onion, chopped
- 2 jalapeño peppers, minced, with or without seeds depending on taste
- 1 tablespoon cumin
- 1 teaspoon minced garlic
- 4½ cups chicken broth or bone broth
- 12 ounces (1½ bricks) cream cheese
- ⅔ cup heavy cream
- 1 teaspoon xanthan gum

1. In a slow cooker, combine the chicken, green chiles, onion, jalapeños, cumin, garlic, and broth.

2. Cook on high for 3 hours. Using two forks, shred the chicken inside the slow cooker.

3. Melt the cream cheese in the microwave. Add it to the slow cooker along with the heavy cream, and stir together. Add the xanthan gum, and stir until well incorporated.

4. Cover, cook for another 30 minutes on high, and serve.

COOKING TIP
Forgot to thaw the chicken? No big deal—just cook for 6 hours on low.

Per Serving (2 cups): Calories: 506; Total Fat: 33g; Carbohydrates: 6.5g; Fiber: 0.5g; Net Carbs: 6g; Protein: 45g; Sugar Alcohols: 0g
Macros: Fat 59% Carbs 5% Protein 36%

Chocolate Whoopie Pies

VEGETARIAN

Prep time: 10 minutes | **Cook time:** 10 minutes | **Servings:** 9

I love cake, and I love cookies, and this is just about the best of both! Whoopie pies are always a huge hit whenever I serve them at a party or bring them somewhere to share. I love chocolate on chocolate, but you can swap the chocolate buttercream for a half-batch of the cream cheese buttercream recipe (page 178).

FOR THE COOKIES

½ cup butter, room temperature

1 cup confectioners' erythritol blend

¼ cup buttermilk

2 large eggs

½ teaspoon vanilla extract

1¼ cups almond flour

¼ cup whey protein isolate, unflavored

2 teaspoons baking powder

¼ teaspoon finely ground black pepper

⅛ teaspoon salt

FOR THE CREAM

2 cup confectioner's erythritol blend

¼ cup unsweetened cocoa powder

¼ cup (½ stick) butter, room temperature

4 ounces (½ brick) cream cheese

½ teaspoon vanilla extract

8 teaspoons boiling water

1. Preheat the oven to 350°F, and line a baking sheet with parchment paper.

2. **To make the cookies:** In a medium bowl with a stand or hand mixer, cream the butter, and then mix in the sweetener, buttermilk, eggs, and vanilla.

3. In a small bowl, sift together the almond flour, whey protein, baking powder, pepper, and salt. Add to the wet mixture, and mix until incorporated. Using a cookie scoop, scoop the dough, use a knife to level the scoop, and place on the lined baking sheet to make 18 cookies.

4. Bake for 9 to 10 minutes, and don't overbake. Remove and set aside to cool.

5. **To make the cream:** In a small bowl stir together the confectioners' sweetener and cocoa powder, and set aside.

6. In a medium bowl, use a stand or hand mixer to cream together the butter, cream cheese, and vanilla. Add the cocoa mixture along with the boiling water, and mix slowly at first and then on high for 1 minute, until completely incorporated.

7. Add the cream mixture to a piping bag or gallon resealable bag with the corner cut off. Flip 9 of the cookies over, pipe the cream evenly on each one, top each one with an additional cookie, and serve. If you don't want to pipe the cream on, use a knife or spoon to put a dollop in the center and press another cookie on top.

SPICE IT UP
Roll the sides in sugar-free chocolate chips, sugar-free sprinkles, or chopped nuts to make them prettier.

Per Serving (1 whoopie pie): Calories: 306; Total Fat: 28g; Carbohydrates: 45g; Fiber: 2.5g; Net Carbs: 2.5g; Protein: 11g; Sugar Alcohols: 40g
Macros: Fat 82% Carbs 3% Protein 14%

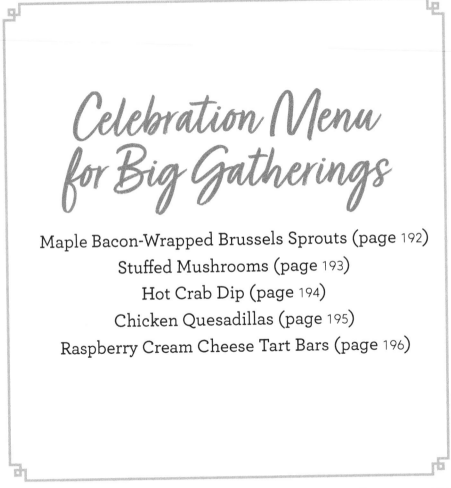

Celebration Menu for Big Gatherings

Maple Bacon-Wrapped Brussels Sprouts (page 192)

Stuffed Mushrooms (page 193)

Hot Crab Dip (page 194)

Chicken Quesadillas (page 195)

Raspberry Cream Cheese Tart Bars (page 196)

Raspberry Cream Cheese Tart Bars, page 196

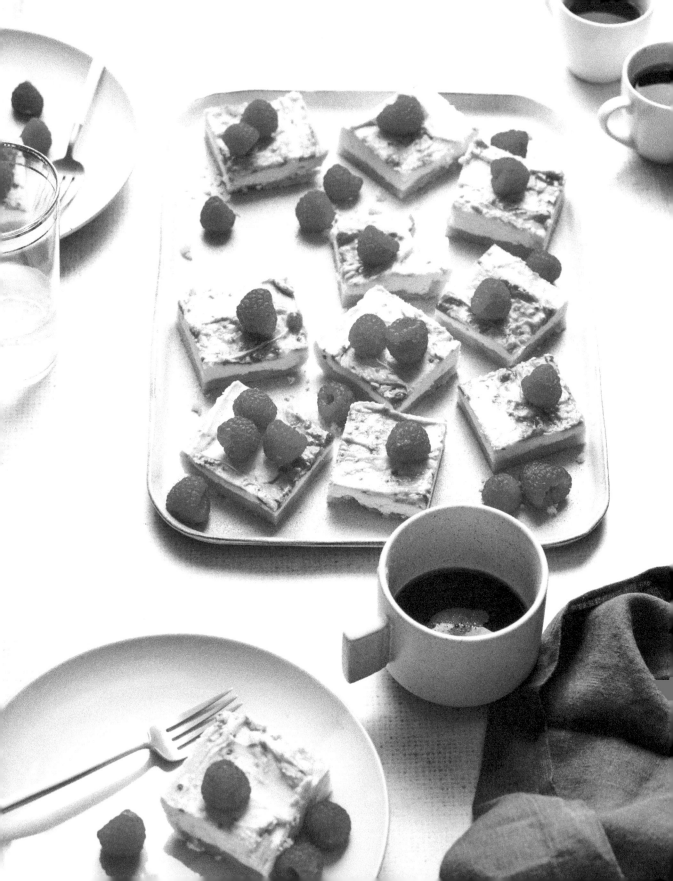

Maple Bacon-Wrapped Brussels Sprouts

DAIRY-FREE, NUT-FREE

Prep time: 10 minutes | **Cook time:** 30 minutes | **Servings:** 20

Whenever I have large parties, I like to serve things that are simple to prepare and easy for folks to eat. This recipe for Brussels sprouts is so yummy, and I'm always asked for the recipe. The sprouts are just fantastic dipped in the spicy maple mayo dip. You could take this recipe up a notch on heat by adding some more sriracha or even a little cayenne pepper, but it's perfect as it is.

20 Brussels sprouts

¾ cup sugar-free maple-flavored syrup, divided

20 slices bacon, cut in half

2 cups mayonnaise

2 teaspoons sriracha sauce

2 teaspoons Dijon mustard

1 teaspoon salt

1 teaspoon freshly ground black pepper

1. Preheat the oven to 400°F, and line a baking sheet with parchment paper.

2. Trim the ends off the Brussels sprouts, remove any wilted leaves, and halve the sprouts lengthwise.

3. Drizzle ¼ cup of syrup on the bacon slices. Roll each Brussels sprout half with a piece of bacon, syrup-side out. Secure with a toothpick, and set them down on the parchment paper, leaving a little room between each sprout.

4. Bake for 30 minutes, or until the bacon is crispy and the Brussels sprouts are fork-tender, rotating the pan halfway through.

5. In a small bowl, mix together the mayonnaise, ½ cup syrup, sriracha, Dijon mustard, salt, and pepper. Serve the Brussels sprouts with the dip.

SWAP IT
Replace the bacon with prosciutto if you'd like.

Per Serving (2 sprouts with dip): Calories: 217; Total Fat: 21g; Carbohydrates: 3.5g; Fiber: 0.5g; Net Carbs: 1.5g; Protein: 5g; Sugar Alcohols: 1.5g
Macros: Fat 87% Carbs 3% Protein 9%

Stuffed Mushrooms

NUT-FREE, VEGETARIAN

Prep time: 20 minutes | **Cook time:** 25 minutes | **Servings:** 20

I remember helping my mother stuff mushroom caps for parties when I was a kid. I always thought it was so fancy and couldn't wait until I got old enough to have a special occasion of my own to make these delicious appetizers. Her recipe was totally keto, so now when I make them, it brings back such beautiful memories of my time in the kitchen with her. They're incredibly tasty and so easy that you can get the mushrooms stuffed and ready to go and then cook them right before your guests arrive.

40 whole fresh white button mushrooms, with rough ends of stems removed

2 tablespoons olive oil

3 garlic cloves, minced

24 ounces (3 bricks) cream cheese, melted

1 cup grated Parmesan cheese

½ teaspoon freshly ground black pepper

½ teaspoon minced onion

½ teaspoon salt

1. Preheat the oven to 375°F, and line a baking sheet with parchment paper.

2. Mince the stems, and place the mushroom caps on the lined baking sheet, stem-side up.

3. In a large skillet over medium heat, heat the olive oil. Place the minced stems in the skillet, and stir for 2 to 3 minutes. Add the garlic, and stir for 30 seconds. Remove from the heat, and stir in the cream cheese, Parmesan, pepper, onion, and salt.

4. With a spoon, fill each mushroom cap with the cheese mixture. Bake for 20 minutes, and serve.

PREP TIP
You could also use a piping bag or resealable bag with the bottom corner cut off to fill the mushroom caps a little faster and make them look fancier.

Per Serving (2 mushrooms): Calories: 145; Total Fat: 13g; Carbohydrates: 4g; Fiber: 0g; Net Carbs: 4g; Protein: 4g; Sugar Alcohols: 0g
Macros: Fat 81% Carbs 11% Protein 11%

Hot Crab Dip

NUT-FREE

Prep time: 10 minutes | **Cook time:** 30 minutes | **Servings:** 20

This warm, cheesy dip is the perfect offering for a large group. With so much flavor, it's also super easy to prepare in advance and then pop in the oven right before company arrives. Offer this savory treat with celery sticks or mushroom halves for dipping, or you could even bake this dip in mushroom caps!

Oil or nonstick cooking spray, for greasing

5 (6-ounce) cans premium lump crabmeat, drained

16 ounces (2 bricks) cream cheese, melted

1 cup sour cream

1 cup mayonnaise

1 cup grated cheddar cheese

1 cup grated mozzarella cheese

2 tablespoons Worcestershire sauce

2 teaspoons garlic powder

1 teaspoon lemon juice

½ teaspoon Tabasco or another hot sauce

1 teaspoon salt

½ teaspoon freshly ground black pepper

Chives, for garnish

1. Preheat the oven to 350°F, and lightly grease a small baking dish.

2. In a large bowl, combine the crabmeat, cream cheese, sour cream, mayonnaise, cheddar, mozzarella, Worcestershire sauce, garlic powder, lemon juice, Tabasco, salt, and pepper, and mix well.

3. Transfer the mixture to the baking dish, and bake for 30 minutes. Garnish with chopped chives, and serve.

PAIR IT
The Garlic Breadsticks made into garlic bread bites (page 165) would be perfect to serve with this dip.

Per Serving: Calories: 246; Total Fat: 22g; Carbohydrates: 2.5g; Fiber: 0g; Net Carbs: 2.5g; Protein: 10g; Sugar Alcohols: 0g
Macros: Fat 80% Carbs 4% Protein 16%

Chicken Quesadillas

NUT-FREE

Prep time: 10 minutes | **Cook time:** 10 minutes | **Servings:** 4

Chicken quesadillas were my son Zack's favorite meal growing up. This treat includes lots of chicken and cheesy greatness topped with sour cream and avocado. A low-carb tortilla (like La Banderita Carb Counter Whole Wheat Wraps) has helped lower the carbs, making this the perfect snack, appetizer, or meal. Here's the basic recipe for your family, but it's super easy to double or even triple, depending on the number of people you're expecting.

2 tablespoons butter

2 tablespoons cream cheese

2 low-carb tortillas

6 ounces grilled chicken, chopped (or canned or rotisserie)

½ cup grated cheddar cheese

½ cup grated mozzarella cheese

2 teaspoons taco seasoning

½ cup sour cream

½ avocado, peeled, pitted, and chopped

1. In a large skillet over medium heat, melt the butter, shifting the pan to spread the butter evenly.

2. Spread the cream cheese evenly on one side of the tortillas. Place one tortilla in the pan, cream cheese–side up. Add the chicken, cheddar, and mozzarella evenly over the tortilla, and season with the taco seasoning. Place the other tortilla on top of the chicken, cream cheese–side down, and cook for 3 to 4 minutes, or until the bottom is golden brown. Carefully flip the tortilla and cook another 3 to 4 minutes, until golden brown.

3. Remove from heat, and allow to cool for a couple of minutes. Slice the quesadilla into 8 wedges, and serve with sour cream and avocado on the side for people to customize their quesadillas.

SWAP IT
Switch up the chicken for ground beef, steak, or even sausage.

Per Serving (2 wedges): Calories: 384; Total Fat: 27g; Carbohydrates: 15g; Fiber: 7g; Net Carbs: 8g; Protein: 21g; Sugar Alcohols: 0g
Macros: Fat 63% Carbs 8% Protein 22%

Raspberry Cream Cheese Tart Bars

VEGETARIAN

Prep time: 10 minutes, plus 1 hour to chill | **Cook time:** 10 minutes | **Servings:** 20

This raspberry cream cheese tart is a showstopper! It's like no-bake cheesecake meets cookie. It's also super easy to make in advance and can be cut into as many servings as you like. For big gatherings, I like to cut 20 bars, but you could easily cut many more or cut the bars larger. We make these all the time, and I know you'll love them, too.

FOR THE COOKIE CRUST

2 cups almond flour

¾ cup confectioners' erythritol blend, sifted

½ teaspoon salt

½ teaspoon baking powder

½ cup (1 stick) cold butter, grated or cubed

FOR THE FILLING

16 ounces (2 bricks) cream cheese, room temperature, cubed

½ cup (1 stick) butter, room temperature, cubed

¼ cup confectioners' erythritol blend, sifted

1 teaspoon vanilla extract

5 tablespoons sugar-free raspberry jam

20 raspberries, for decoration

1. Preheat the oven to 350°F, and line a 9-by-13-inch pan with parchment paper so it sticks out over the top on at least two sides.

2. **To make the cookie crust:** Stir together the almond flour, confectioners' sweetener, salt, and baking powder. Add the butter, and with your fingers, work the ingredients together until completely incorporated. It will be crumbly.

3. Transfer the dough into the pan, and distribute evenly, using your fingers to mash down all over until it's smooth and completely covering the bottom of the pan.

4. Bake for 10 to 14 minutes, or until golden brown on top, rotating the pan halfway through.

5. **To make the filling:** In a large bowl, combine the cream cheese, butter, confectioners' sweetener, and vanilla. Using a mixer, whip on high for 2 minutes until completely smooth.

6. Place the jam in a microwave-safe dish, and microwave for about 20 seconds, just long enough to get it smooth. Pour the jam into the cream cheese mixture, and fold together just until it has a marbled look.

7. When the crust has cooled, spoon the cream cheese mixture on top, and spread evenly. Cover and refrigerate for at least an hour. Remove from the refrigerator, and use the overhanging parchment paper to lift the tart out of the pan and onto the counter. Cut the tart into 20 bars, top each one with a raspberry, and place on a tray to serve.

SWAP IT

I chose raspberry for this recipe, but you could choose any flavor of sugar-free jam you like. You could also split the cream cheese mixture in half or thirds, add to each whatever flavors of jam you like, and have a variety.

Per Serving (1 bar): Calories: 220; Total Fat: 22g; Carbohydrates: 10.5g; Fiber: 2g; Net Carbs: 2.5g; Protein: 4g; Sugar Alcohols: 6g
Macros: Fat 90% Carbs 5% Protein 7%

CHAPTER EIGHT

Cocktails for All Seasons

You don't have to give up cocktails completely on keto! Just make a few adjustments here and there to make them more keto-friendly. In this section, you'll find some of my favorite fresh, warm-weather recipes for spring and summer as well as fall and winter specialties perfect for chilly nights and special toasts. No matter what time of year, you'll enjoy them all! And perhaps this goes without saying, but feel free to adjust the alcohol amounts to your liking. I can't help it—I like a stiff drink!

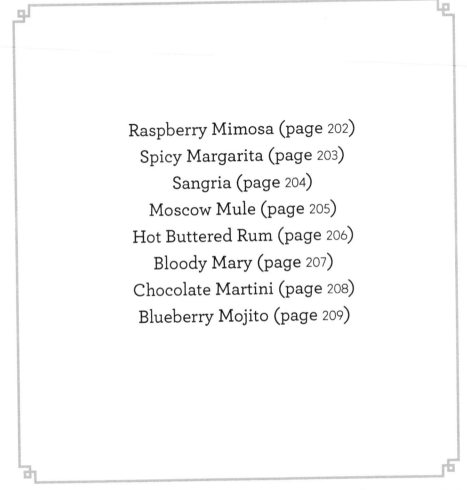

Raspberry Mimosa, page 202

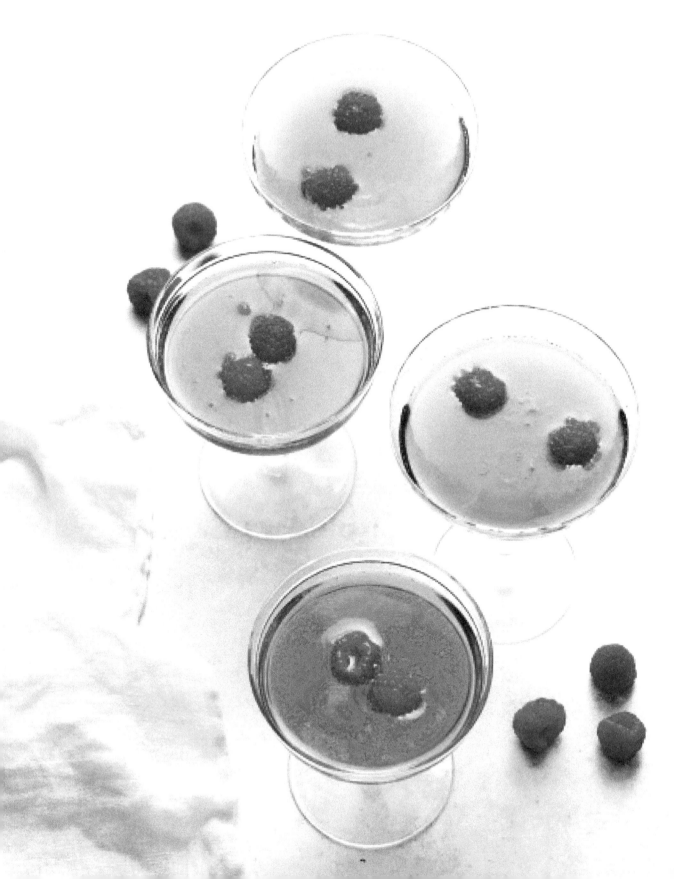

Raspberry Mimosa

DAIRY-FREE, NUT-FREE, VEGAN

Prep time: 10 minutes | **Cook time:** 5 minutes | **Servings:** 4

There's something about a mimosa, with the orange juice and champagne in a long flute, that's just so fancy and delicious served on Easter morning, at brunch, or any other time. I decided to put a twist on this cocktail and try raspberry instead of orange to make it a little more keto-friendly. The pink raspberry makes it a work of art, but you could use any other berries as well. When you're shopping for the champagne, look for brut, extra brut, or extra dry. Any of these will be great and under 2 carbs per 6-ounce serving. Brut naturally has the fewest carbs, if you can find it.

6 ounces raspberries (roughly 28 raspberries), divided

2 tablespoons granulated erythritol blend
¼ cup water

1 bottle brut or dry champagne
Mint leaves, for garnish

1. In a small saucepan over medium heat, add 20 raspberries, the sweetener, and the water. Continue to stir occasionally until the berries break down, 3 to 4 minutes.

2. Remove from the heat, pour into a blender, and pulse 6 to 8 times. Pour the mixture into a strainer to remove all the seeds. Use the back of a spoon to push the mixture through the strainer.

3. Add a few tablespoons of the raspberry mixture to a champagne glass, pour 6 ounces of champagne on top, and stir. Drop two of the remaining raspberries into each glass, add mint for garnish, and serve.

SERVING TIP
To be extra fancy, you could roll the raspberries for garnish in a little bit of granulated sweetener and perch them on the edge of the glasses instead of dropping them into the drinks. Looks very pretty!

Per Serving: Calories: 178; Total Fat: 0g; Carbohydrates: 16g; Fiber: 3g; Net Carbs: 7g; Protein: 1g; Sugar Alcohols: 6g
Macros: Fat 0% Carbs 16% Protein 2%

Spicy Margarita

DAIRY-FREE, NUT-FREE, VEGAN

Prep time: 10 minutes | **Servings:** 4

A good margarita reminds me of sitting on a patio with friends on a sunny day with lots of laughter and good memories to follow. I'm an "on the rocks girl," but you could easily pour this recipe over ice in a blender and serve the drinks up frozen. Cinco de Mayo or Taco Tuesday, every day is Margarita Day in my book!

¼ cup kosher salt, for garnish

½ cup freshly squeezed lime juice, plus 4 small slices for garnish

Ice

8 ounces tequila

¼ cup freshly squeezed orange juice

12 drops liquid stevia, plus more if needed

1 jalapeño, thinly sliced, with or without seeds depending on taste

1. Place the salt on a shallow plate. Using one of the limes, rub the rims of four glasses. Dip the glasses in the salt, and then carefully add some ice to each glass.

2. Combine the tequila, lime juice, orange juice, stevia, and jalapeño slices and a few ice cubes in a shaker or Mason jar, and shake vigorously. Taste, add a few more drops of stevia if needed, and then pour evenly into the glasses.

3. Garnish each glass edge with a lime slice, and serve.

SERVING TIP
You can add a little more heat to this drink by adding more jalapeño or jalapeño juice from a jar. To lighten it up, add some sugar-free/diet ginger ale.

Per Serving: Calories: 143; Total Fat: 0g; Carbohydrates: 4g; Fiber: 0g; Net Carbs: 4g; Protein: 0g; Sugar Alcohols: 0g
Macros: Fat 0% Carbs 11% Protein 0%

Sangria

DAIRY-FREE, NUT-FREE, VEGAN

Prep time: 15 minutes, plus 2 hours to chill | **Servings:** 6

Sangria reminds me of my trip to Spain, where I tasted so many versions as I traveled throughout the country. From what I remember on my tour, sangria originated back in the Middle Ages when the water was unsafe to drink. It's such a refreshing drink, especially on a hot summer day—fruity and festive with Mexican food or perfect with a charcuterie tray full of all your favorite meats, cheeses, nuts, and olives. It's better to make this and let it marinate for 6 to 8 hours, but you could also whip it up and serve it right away.

1 bottle Pinot Noir, preferably Spanish

¼ cup freshly squeezed orange juice, plus 2 slices cut in quarters, for garnish

⅓ cup sliced strawberries

⅓ cup blueberries

1 small lemon, thinly sliced

1 or 2 tablespoons sugar-free maple-flavored syrup

½ cup brandy

1. In a pitcher, mix the wine, orange juice, strawberries, blueberries, lemon slices, syrup, and brandy.
2. Refrigerate for 2 to 8 hours, stirring occasionally.
3. Pour in a glass over a small amount of ice, garnish the side of the glass with an orange quarter, and serve.

SERVING TIP
If you want to lighten it up, add a little fizz, or stretch the amount of servings of your sangria, try adding ½ cup of club soda.

Per Serving: Calories: 160; Total Fat: 0g; Carbohydrates: 7g; Fiber: 0.5g; Net Carbs: 5.5g; Protein: 0g; Sugar Alcohols: 1g
Macros: Fat 0% Carbs 14% Protein 0%

Moscow Mule

DAIRY-FREE, NUT-FREE, VEGAN

Prep time: 5 minutes | **Servings:** 4

The Moscow Mule is such a refreshing summertime drink. There's even something so fun about the copper cup that keeps it cold and makes it look super festive. For this recipe, you certainly don't need the copper cups, but somehow Moscow Mules do taste better from those pretty cups! Guests always want the recipe and are thrilled when they hear how easy it is.

Ice

8 ounces vodka

¼ cup freshly squeezed lime juice (about 2 limes),

reserving a slice to quarter, for garnish

16 ounces sugar-free ginger beer

Mint leaves, for garnish

1. Add crushed ice or cubes to four copper cups or cocktail glasses.

2. In a shaker or Mason jar, add the vodka and lime juice, along with a few ice cubes, and shake. Pour over ice in glasses. Pour 4 ounces of ginger beer in each glass, and stir.

3. Add a lime quarter to each glass, garnish with mint, and serve.

SWAP IT

If you can't find a sugar-free ginger beer (like Gosling's), you can always use sugar-free ginger ale.

Per Serving: Calories: 168; Total Fat: 0g; Carbohydrates: 1g; Fiber: 0g; Net Carbs: 1g; Protein: 0g; Sugar Alcohols: 0g
Macros: Fat 0% Carbs 2% Protein 0%

Hot Buttered Rum

NUT-FREE, VEGETARIAN

Prep time: 5 minutes | **Cook time:** 5 minutes | **Servings:** 4

There are not enough yummy words to describe how good this hot buttered rum is. I've always been a huge fan of cuddling up with a warm cup and watching holiday movies or enjoying the fire on cold winter nights. It's so romantic for two, but you could also impress a lot of guests with this as a nightcap to a perfect evening. Served warm is my preference, but you could also drop this over some ice in a blender and serve it cold on a sunny day.

½ cup butter

¾ cup brown erythritol blend

¼ cup sugar-free maple-flavored syrup

½ teaspoon pumpkin pie spice

Pinch salt

2 cups water

8 ounces spiced rum

4 cinnamon sticks, for garnish

1. In a medium saucepan over medium heat, add the butter, brown sweetener, syrup, pumpkin pie spice, salt, and water, and stir until completely melted and incorporated, 3 to 4 minutes.

2. Remove from the heat, add the rum, pour evenly into four mugs, garnish each with a cinnamon stick, stir, and serve.

SERVING TIP
Add a dollop of sugar-free whipped cream (page 114) topped with a sprinkle of cinnamon to dress this drink up even more.

Per Serving: Calories: 341; Total Fat: 23g; Carbohydrates: 38g; Fiber: 0g; Net Carbs: 0g; Protein: 0g; Sugar Alcohols: 38g
Macros: Fat 61% Carbs 0% Protein 0%

Bloody Mary

NUT-FREE

Prep time: 5 minutes | **Servings:** 6

I hosted a "Bloody Mary Bar Party" that centered on this cocktail, and it was great. I made this basic recipe and set out all kinds of outrageous garnishes for guests to choose from and add to their drink, and then we voted on who made the craziest version. Basically, anything you serve on a charcuterie board would make for perfect garnishes. Just make sure to have lots of bamboo skewers for all your creations!

FOR THE BLOODY MARY
1 (32-ounce) bottle V8 Juice, original or spicy
5 teaspoons Worcestershire sauce
1 tablespoon prepared horseradish
¼ teaspoon freshly ground black pepper

1 teaspoon garlic salt
1 teaspoon celery salt
2 teaspoons sriracha sauce
Ice
12 ounces vodka

FOR THE GLASS RIM
1 tablespoon celery salt
1 tablespoon kosher salt
1 lime, cut into wedges

FOR GARNISH
6 celery stalks, ends cut off, leaves remaining
6 slices crispy bacon
12 blue cheese–stuffed olives, or your favorite

1. In a large pitcher, mix together the V8 Juice, Worcestershire sauce, horse-radish, pepper, garlic salt, celery salt, and sriracha. Refrigerate until ready to serve.

2. In a shallow plate, mix the celery salt and kosher salt for the glass rims. Using one wedge of lime, rub the rims of eight (10-ounce) glasses, and then dip them into the salt mixture.

3. Carefully fill each glass with ice, trying not to disturb the salt on the rim, and pour 2 ounces of vodka into each glass. Pour the tomato mixture over each glass, and garnish with a stalk of celery and piece of bacon.

4. Skewer two olives on a bamboo skewer and place across the top, garnish the edge of the glass with a lime wedge or just add to the glass, and serve.

Per Serving: Calories: 256; Total Fat: 7.5g; Carbohydrates: 9g; Fiber: 1.5g; Net Carbs: 7.5g; Protein: 5g; Sugar Alcohols: 0g
Macros: Fat 26% Carbs 12% Protein 8%

Chocolate Martini

VEGETARIAN

Prep time: 10 minutes | **Servings:** 4

Chocolate martini? Uh, yes please! Anything chocolate is all right with me, especially when it's mixed with vodka. I use the chocolate sauce from my Churros and Chocolate Sauce (page 54)—really you can use that sauce on anything from keto pancakes to a bowl of berries and whipped cream. This drink is so velvety smooth. Add a little peppermint extract to make it even more special for the winter holidays.

½ chocolate sauce recipe (page 54), divided

8 ounces vodka

1 cup half-and-half

Ice

1. Drizzle 1 teaspoon of chocolate sauce around the edges of four chilled martini glasses.

2. In a shaker or Mason jar with a lid, add the rest of the chocolate sauce, vodka, half-and-half, and ice cubes, and shake for at least 30 seconds. Pour into the glasses, straining out the ice cubes, and serve.

SPICE IT UP
A little heat will intensify the taste of the chocolate and take this drink to a whole new level—just add a bit of cayenne pepper!

Per Serving: Calories: 268; Total Fat: 12g; Carbohydrates: 14g; Fiber: 2g; Net Carbs: 4.5g; Protein: 3g; Sugar Alcohols: 7.5g
Macros: Fat 40% Carbs 7% Protein 4%

Blueberry Mojito

DAIRY-FREE, NUT-FREE, VEGAN

Prep time: 10 minutes | **Servings:** 4

I discovered this cocktail while on vacation in Mexico. The addition of blueberries is such a different twist on the traditional mojito. It's light and refreshing and makes such a beautiful presentation. It's perfect for any time of year, but especially in the summer when you're sitting out by the pool with friends.

½ cup granulated erythritol blend, plus more for the rims

2 limes, half of one cut into 8 lime wheel slices for garnish

Ice

¾ cup fresh blueberries, divided

3 tablespoons fresh lime juice

4 large mint leaves torn in pieces, and extra leaves for garnish

8 ounces white rum

1-liter bottle club soda

1. Place a little sweetener on a shallow plate. Rub the rim of four (10-ounce) chilled glass tumblers with lime and dip the rims into the sweetener. Add ice cubes, being careful not to disturb the sugar rim.

2. In a shaker or Mason jar with a lid, add ½ cup of blueberries, sweetener, lime juice, and mint leaves. Muddle using the back of a wooden spoon or a muddler.

3. Add the rum and some ice to the jar, and shake for at least 45 seconds. Pour over the ice in the glasses, fill with club soda, and stir. Drop a lime wheel in the glass and one on the rim for garnish, drop the remaining blueberries equally into each glass, and serve.

SERVING TIP
You can also roll a few of the blueberries in sugar, skewer them, and place across each of the glasses.

Per Serving: Calories: 148; Total Fat: 0g; Carbohydrates: 29g; Fiber: 0.5g; Net Carbs: 4.5g; Protein: 0g; Sugar Alcohols: 24g
Macros: Fat 0% Carbs 12% Protein 0%

Resources

Visit my Instagram page at @ketohabits! Here are some more resources that I have found invaluable on my journey:

@cheftaffyelrod: For more keto inspiration, visit my friend and fellow keto chef Taffy Elrod for additional keto tips and ideas.

charliefoundation.org: The Charlie Foundation for Ketogenic Therapies, founded in 1994, provides information about diet therapies for people with epilepsy, other neurological disorders, and select cancers. You will find so much information on this site.

perfectketo.com: Founded by Dr. Anthony Gustin, Perfect Keto focuses on improving health by providing products that help you reach your goals. I have used its MCT Oil Powder and Collagen Powder in my coffee every single morning since I started this lifestyle, and I love its snack bars as well. Its website is a wealth of information with articles, recipes, and an online macro calculator. You can find the Perfect Keto macro calculator at perfectketo.com/keto-macro-calculator.

mariamindbodyhealth.com: Maria Emmerich is a nutritionist who specializes in the ketogenic diet and exercise physiology. Her book *Keto* is a wealth of information, and she has written many cookbooks as well. You can find her macro calculator at mariamindbodyhealth.com/keto-calculator.

cutdacarb.com: These wraps are a staple at our house. We make pizza, tortilla chips, and so much more with them. They are amazing.

gooddees.com: It's fun to bake goodies at home, and if you want some delicious mixes with great ingredients, this is where you go!

kettleandfire.com: The best bone broths and keto soups available.

keto-mojo.com: I have used its Keto-Mojo for ketone/glucose testing for years and am a huge fan.

dropanfbomb.com: Also a staple at our house, FBombs are the best-quality fats in a form that is easy to carry, use, and enjoy.

Index

211

Acknowledgments

I would first of all like to thank my son Zack for all of his love, support, and patience with all the technical assistance regarding this book. I couldn't have done it without you. Also, my father, who has always backed me up, been on my side, and encouraged me to be the best I can be. A big thank you as well to Ada Fung and all the folks at Callisto Media, who have given me the chance, once again, to "shine." And to David, my "Lovies," the love of my life. God surely saved the best for last when he led me to you.

About the Author

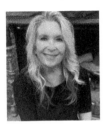 Mary Alexander is the author of the popular Instagram account @KetoHabits, which she started in early 2016 for, as she puts it, "accountability." She decided something had to change, weight and health wise, after seeing herself in a bathing suit picture while on vacation. On Valentine's Day 2016, she started the ketogenic lifestyle with her partner, David (referred to always as "Lovies"). Mary has lost over 60 pounds with keto and enjoys baking, blogging, and inspiring all who follow her to embrace how easy, effective, and life-changing keto can be. As the retired owner of Mary Alexander Cakes, she brings a lot to the table with a growing list of delicious recipes that she has "keto-fied." Her before-and-after keto accomplishments were featured in a *Reader's Digest* article.

Mary lives in Texas with Lovies, and together they share three beautiful children, Zack, Kristina, and Chris. They enjoy family challenges and collectively have lost almost 200 pounds.